Dermatoscopy in Clinical Practice

Series in Dermatological Treatment

Series editors

Steven R Feldman

and

Peter van de Kerkhof

Published in association with the *Journal of Dermatological Treatment*

1. Robert Baran, Roderick Hay, Eckhart Haneke, Antonella Tosti
   Onychomycosis, second edition, ISBN 9780415385794
2. Ronald Marks
   Facial Skin Disorders, ISBN 9781841842103
3. Sakari Reitamo, Thomas Luger, Martin Steinhoff
   Textbook of Atopic Dermatitis, ISBN 9781841842462
4. Calum C Lyon, Amanda J Smith
   Abdominal Stomas and Their Skin Disorders, Second Edition, ISBN 9781841844312
5. Leonard Goldberg
   Atlas of Flaps of the Face, ISBN 9781853177262
6. Antonella Tosti, Maria Pia De Padova, Kenneth Beer
   Acne Scars: Classification and Treatment, ISBN 9781841846873
7. Bertrand Richert, Nilton di Chiacchio, Eckart Haneke
   Nail Surgery, ISBN 9780415472333
8. Giuseppe Micali, Francesco Lacarrubba
   Dermatoscopy in Clinical Practice: Beyond Pigmented Lesions, ISBN 9780415468732

Dermatoscopy in Clinical Practice
Beyond Pigmented Lesions
Second Edition

Edited by
Giuseppe Micali, MD
and
Francesco Lacarrubba, MD
Dermatology Clinic
University of Catania, Italy

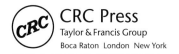

CRC Press
Taylor & Francis Group
Boca Raton London New York

CRC Press is an imprint of the
Taylor & Francis Group, an **informa** business

CRC Press
Taylor & Francis Group
6000 Broken Sound Parkway NW, Suite 300
Boca Raton, FL 33487-2742

© 2016 by Taylor & Francis Group, LLC
CRC Press is an imprint of Taylor & Francis Group, an Informa business

No claim to original U.S. Government works

Printed and bound in India by Replika Press Pvt. Ltd.

Printed on acid-free paper
Version Date: 20151211

International Standard Book Number-13: 978-1-4822-2595-2 (Hardback)

This book contains information obtained from authentic and highly regarded sources. While all reasonable efforts have been made to publish reliable data and information, neither the author[s] nor the publisher can accept any legal responsibility or liability for any errors or omissions that may be made. The publishers wish to make clear that any views or opinions expressed in this book by individual editors, authors or contributors are personal to them and do not necessarily reflect the views/opinions of the publishers. The information or guidance contained in this book is intended for use by medical, scientific or health-care professionals and is provided strictly as a supplement to the medical or other professional's own judgement, their knowledge of the patient's medical history, relevant manufacturer's instructions and the appropriate best practice guidelines. Because of the rapid advances in medical science, any information or advice on dosages, procedures or diagnoses should be independently verified. The reader is strongly urged to consult the relevant national drug formulary and the drug companies' and device or material manufacturers' printed instructions, and their websites, before administering or utilizing any of the drugs, devices or materials mentioned in this book. This book does not indicate whether a particular treatment is appropriate or suitable for a particular individual. Ultimately it is the sole responsibility of the medical professional to make his or her own professional judgements, so as to advise and treat patients appropriately. The authors and publishers have also attempted to trace the copyright holders of all material reproduced in this publication and apologize to copyright holders if permission to publish in this form has not been obtained. If any copyright material has not been acknowledged please write and let us know so we may rectify in any future reprint.

Except as permitted under U.S. Copyright Law, no part of this book may be reprinted, reproduced, transmitted, or utilized in any form by any electronic, mechanical, or other means, now known or hereafter invented, including photocopying, microfilming, and recording, or in any information storage or retrieval system, without written permission from the publishers.

For permission to photocopy or use material electronically from this work, please access www.copyright.com (http://www.copyright.com/) or contact the Copyright Clearance Center, Inc. (CCC), 222 Rosewood Drive, Danvers, MA 01923, 978-750-8400. CCC is a not-for-profit organization that provides licenses and registration for a variety of users. For organizations that have been granted a photocopy license by the CCC, a separate system of payment has been arranged.

Trademark Notice: Product or corporate names may be trademarks or registered trademarks, and are used only for identification and explanation without intent to infringe.

Library of Congress Cataloging-in-Publication Data

Names: Micali, Giuseppe, editor. | Lacarrubba, Francesco, editor.
Title: Dermatoscopy in clinical practice : beyond pigmented lesions / [edited by] Giuseppe Micali, Francesco Lacarrubba.
Description: Second edition. | Boca Raton : Taylor & Francis, 2016. |
Includes bibliographical references and index.
Identifiers: LCCN 2015048582| ISBN 9781482225952 (hardback : alk. paper) |
ISBN 9781482225990 (e-book)
Subjects: | MESH: Dermoscopy--methods | Skin Diseases--diagnosis | Atlases
Classification: LCC RL96 | NLM WR 17 | DDC 616.5/0757--dc23
LC record available at http://lccn.loc.gov/2015048582

Visit the Taylor & Francis Web site at
http://www.taylorandfrancis.com

and the CRC Press Web site at
http://www.crcpress.com

Contents

Introduction xi
List of contributors xiii

1 Equipment for dermatoscopy/videodermatoscopy 1

Pietro Rubegni, Niccolò Nami, Luca Feci, Marco Burroni, Linda Tognetti, and Michele Fimiani

Dermatoscopy 1
Videodermatoscopy 1
Data storage 3
Software for objective assessment and assisted diagnosis 3
Conclusions 5
References 6

2 Parasitoses: Scabies 9

Giuseppe Micali, Francesco Lacarrubba, and Robert A. Schwartz

Definition 9
Epidemiology/Etiopathogenesis 9
Clinical presentation/Diagnosis 9
Dermatoscopy/Videodermatoscopy features 10
References 14

3 Parasitoses: Pediculosis 15

Francesco Lacarrubba, Giuseppe Micali, Alessandro Di Stefani, and Robert A. Schwartz

Head lice 15
Crab lice 17
References 19

4 Parasitoses: Therapeutic monitoring of scabies and pediculosis 21

Giuseppe Micali, Aurora Tedeschi, Francesco Lacarrubba, and Dennis P. West

Therapeutic monitoring of scabies 21
Therapeutic monitoring of pediculosis 24
References 26

5 Parasitoses: Tungiasis 27

Elvira Moscarella, Leonardo Spagnol Abraham, and Giuseppe Argenziano

Definition 27
Epidemiology/Etiopathogenesis 27
Clinical presentation/Diagnosis 27
Dermatoscopy/Videodermatoscopy features 28
References 29

6 Parasitoses: Cutaneous larva migrans ... 31

Elvira Moscarella, Renato Bakos, and Giuseppe Argenziano
Definition ... 31
Epidemiology/Etiopathogenesis ... 31
Clinical presentation/Diagnosis ... 31
Dermatoscopy/Videodermatoscopy features ... 31
References ... 32

7 Parasitoses: Cutaneous leishmaniasis ... 33

Pedro Zaballos Diego
Definition ... 33
Epidemiology/Etiopathogenesis ... 33
Clinical presentation/Diagnosis ... 33
Dermatoscopy/Videodermatoscopy features ... 33
References ... 35

8 Parasitoses: Trombiculiasis ... 37

Maria Rita Nasca and Giuseppe Micali
Definition ... 37
Epidemiology/Etiopathogenesis ... 37
Clinical presentation/Diagnosis ... 37
Dermatoscopy/Videodermatoscopy features ... 37
References ... 38

9 Infectious diseases: Cutaneous and genital warts ... 39

Francesco Lacarrubba, Anna Elisa Verzì, Marco Ardigò, and Giuseppe Micali
Cutaneous warts ... 39
Genital warts ... 41
References ... 42

10 Infectious diseases: Molluscum contagiosum ... 43

Pedro Zaballos Diego
Definition ... 43
Epidemiology/Etiopathogenesis ... 43
Clinical presentation/Diagnosis ... 43
Dermatoscopy/Videodermatoscopy features ... 43
References ... 45

11 Infectious diseases: Tinea capitis ... 47

Saleh El-Shiemy, Hoda Monieb, Wael Saudi, and Sara Mohy
Definition ... 47
Epidemiology/Etiopathogenesis ... 47
Clinical presentation/Diagnosis ... 47
Dermatoscopy/Videodermatoscopy features ... 47
References ... 52

12 Hair loss and hair shaft disorders 55

Antonella Tosti
Normal scalp 55
Androgenetic alopecia 55
Alopecia areata 55
Alopecia areata incognita 57
Trichotillomania 58
Congenital triangular alopecia 58
Scarring alopecia 58
Hair shaft disorders 62
References 66

13 Inflammatory diseases: Psoriasis 67

Francesco Lacarrubba, Giorgio Filosa, Rossella De Angelis, Leonardo Bugatti, Maria Concetta Potenza, Ilaria Proietti, Robert A. Schwartz, Maria Letizia Musumeci, Maria Rita Nasca, Paolo Rosina, and Giuseppe Micali
Definition 67
Epidemiology/Etiopathogenesis 67
Clinical presentation/Diagnosis 67
Dermatoscopy/Videodermatoscopy features 69
Therapeutic monitoring of psoriasis 76
References 77

14 Inflammatory diseases: Lichen planus 79

Francisco Vázquez-López and Felipe Valdes Pineda
Definition 79
Epidemiology/Etiopathogenesis 79
Clinical presentation/Diagnosis 79
Dermatoscopy/Videodermatoscopy features 80
References 84

15 Inflammatory diseases: Common urticaria and urticarial vasculitis 87

Francisco Vázquez-López and Felipe Valdes Pineda
Definition 87
Epidemiology/Etiopathogenesis 87
Clinical presentation/Diagnosis 87
Dermatoscopy/Videodermatoscopy features 88
References 91

16 Inflammatory diseases: Connective tissue diseases 93

Paolo Rosina
Definition 93
Epidemiology/Etiopathogenesis 93
Clinical presentation/Diagnosis 93
Dermatoscopy/Videodermatoscopy features 93
References 96

17 Inflammatory diseases: Rosacea 97

Paolo Rosina
Definition 97
Epidemiology/Etiopathogenesis 97
Clinical presentation/Diagnosis 97
Dermatoscopy/Videodermatoscopy features 97
References 99

18 Inflammatory diseases: Pigmented purpuric dermatoses 101

Pedro Zaballos Diego
Definition 101
Epidemiology/Etiopathogenesis 101
Clinical presentation/Diagnosis 101
Dermatoscopy/Videodermatoscopy features 101
References 103

19 Inflammatory diseases: Pityriasis lichenoides 105

Giuseppe Stinco, Francesco Lacarrubba, Enzo Errichetti, and Giuseppe Micali
Definition 105
Epidemiology/Etiopathogenesis 105
Clinical presentation/Diagnosis 105
Dermatoscopy/Videodermatoscopy features 106
References 108

20 Inflammatory diseases: Granulomatous skin disorders and Wolf's isotopic response lesions 111

Francisco Vázquez-López, Celia Gómez de Castro, and Noemi Eiris-Salvado
Granulomatous skin disorders 111
Wolf's isotopic response lesions 114
References 115

21 Nonpigmented skin lesions: Clear cell acanthoma 117

Francesco Lacarrubba, Federica Dall'Oglio, and Giuseppe Micali
Definition 117
Epidemiology/Etiopathogenesis 117
Clinical presentation/Diagnosis 117
Dermatoscopy/Videodermatoscopy features 117
References 119

22 Nonpigmented skin lesions: Pyogenic granuloma 121

Pedro Zaballos Diego
Definition 121
Epidemiology/Etiopathogenesis 121
Clinical presentation/Diagnosis 121
Dermatoscopy/Videodermatoscopy features 121
References 124

Contents

23 Nonpigmented skin lesions: Angiokeratoma **125**

Anna Elisa Verzì, Francesco Lacarrubba, and Giuseppe Micali
Definition 125
Epidemiology/Etiopathogenesis 125
Clinical presentation/Diagnosis 125
Dermatoscopy/Videodermatoscopy features 125
References 126

24 Nonpigmented skin lesions: Sebaceous hyperplasia **127**

Pedro Zaballos Diego
Definition 127
Epidemiology/Etiopathogenesis 127
Clinical presentation/Diagnosis 127
Dermatoscopy/Videodermatoscopy features 127
References 129

25 Nonpigmented skin lesions: Xanthomatous lesions **131**

Pietro Rubegni, Linda Tognetti, Filomena Mandato, and Michele Fimiani
Definition 131
Epidemiology/Etiopathogenesis 131
Clinical presentation/Diagnosis 131
Dermatoscopy/Videodermatoscopy features 133
References 135

26 Nonpigmented skin lesions: Porokeratosis **137**

Pedro Zaballos Diego
Definition 137
Epidemiology/Etiopathogenesis 137
Clinical presentation/Diagnosis 137
Dermatoscopy/Videodermatoscopy features 137
References 139

27 Nonpigmented skin lesions: Apocrine hidrocystoma **141**

Pedro Zaballos Diego
Definition 141
Epidemiology/Etiopathogenesis 141
Clinical presentation/Diagnosis 141
Dermatoscopy/Videodermatoscopy features 141
References 143

28 Nonpigmented skin lesions: Bowen's disease **145**

Leonardo Bugatti and Giorgio Filosa
Definition 145
Epidemiology/Etiopathogenesis 145
Clinical presentation/Diagnosis 145
Dermatoscopy/Videodermatoscopy features 146
References 149

29 Nonpigmented skin lesions: Actinic keratosis and squamous cell carcinoma .. 151

Aimilios Lallas and Giuseppe Argenziano

Actinic keratosis 151
Squamous cell carcinoma 154
References 156

30 Capillary malformations 159

Francisco Vazquez-Lopez and Begoña García-García

Definition 159
Epidemiology/Etiopathogenesis 159
Clinical presentation/Diagnosis 159
Dermatoscopy/Videodermatoscopy features 160
References 164

31 Miscellaneous disorders 167

Enzo Errichetti, Giuseppe Stinco, Anna Elisa Verzì, Francesco Lacarrubba, Salvatore Ferraro, Cecilia Santagati, and Giuseppe Micali

Lichen sclerosus 167
Morphea 168
Lichen nitidus 169
Darier's disease 170
Fordyce's spots of the penile shaft 171
Pearly penile papules and vestibular papillae 172
Kaposi's sarcoma 173
Cutaneous mastocytosis 174
Milia 176
References 177

32 Photodamaged and aged skin 179

Anne-Sophie Brillouet and Michael D. Southall

Dermatoscopy and skin glyphics 179
Skin microglyphics as a function of aging 179
Evaluating skin glyphic changes with emollient treatment 181
Role of skin glyphics as a reservoir for emollients and other topical agents 183
Conclusion 183
References 183

Index 185

Introduction

Dermatoscopy (D), also called "dermoscopy" or "incident light microscopy," is a noninvasive technique that allows rapid and magnified *in vivo* observation of the skin with the visualization of morphologic features that are invisible to the naked eye. It may be performed with manual devices that do not require any computer assistance, and allow magnifications up to ×10, or with digital systems requiring a video camera equipped with optic fibers and lenses that ensure magnifications of up to ×1000; in the latter instance the term videodermatoscopy (VD) is used. The images obtained are visualized on a monitor and stored on a personal computer in order to process them and compare any possible changes over time. In many ways, VD represents the evolution of D. In this book the term *dermatoscopy* refers to the use of manual devices and *videodermatoscopy* to the use of digital systems operating at high magnifications.

In the past, new terms such as trichoscopy, entodermoscopy, and inflammoscopy, that address specific applications (hair, skin parasitoses, inflammatory disorders, etc.), have appeared in scientific articles.

Both D and VD are widely used in the differential diagnosis of pigmented skin lesions, usually through *epiluminescence microscopy*, which involves the application of a liquid (oil, alcohol, or water) to the skin to eliminate light reflection; however, systems utilizing polarized light may achieve similar results without the need for liquids. In addition to their most common use for the differential diagnosis of pigmented skin lesions, it has been demonstrated that D/VD have expanded applications in dermatology. Alternative applications of D/VD include inflammatory diseases, parasitoses, hair and nail abnormalities, and a large variety of other dermatologic conditions, as well as cosmetology. For many of these disorders the use of high magnification is needed for research as well as for clinical purposes. Depending on the skin disorder, D/VD may be useful for differential diagnosis, prognostic evaluation, and monitoring response to treatment. The capability to capture digital images is perfectly suited to teledermatology—the "store-and-forward" technique that allows the exchange of opinions between dermatologists—and might be useful when on-site D/VD services are not available.

The aim of this book is to advance knowledge of enhanced visualization/digital imaging using D or VD beyond the traditional indication of pigmented lesions of the skin. The focus is on conditions in which these techniques are most useful, describing the clinical and histopathological correlations associated with the procedure. The numerous images provided will be useful in the daily clinical practice of dermatologists, who should thus be encouraged to utilize D/VD in the routine evaluation of skin diseases. The book is an important yet relatively simple addition to the dermatologist's daily office practice.

Contributors

Marco Ardigò
Department of Clinical Dermatology
San Gallicano Dermatological Institute
Rome, Italy

Giuseppe Argenziano
Dermatology Unit
Second University of Naples, Italy

Renato Bakos
Department of Dermatology
Hospital de Clínicas de Porto Alegre
Universidade Federal do Rio Grande do Sul
Porto Alegre, Brazil

Anne-Sophie Brillouet
Johnson & Johnson Skin Research Center
CPPW
Johnson & Johnson Consumer Companies Inc.
Skillman, New Jersey, USA

Leonardo Bugatti
Dermatology Unit "Carlo Urbani" Hospital
Jesi, Italy

Marco Burroni
Department of Medical Science
Surgery and Neuroscience
Section of Dermatology
University of Siena, Italy

Federica Dall'Oglio
Dermatology Clinic
University of Catania, Italy

Rossella De Angelis
Dermatology Unit "Carlo Urbani" Hospital
Jesi, Italy

Alessandro Di Stefani
Division of Dermatology
Complesso Integrato Columbus
Catholic University of the Sacred Heart
Rome, Italy

Noemi Eiris-Salvado
Department of Dermatology
Hospital Universitario Central de Asturias
Oviedo, Asturias, Spain

Saleh El-Shiemy
Ain Shams University and Misr University for
Science and Technology (MUST), Egypt

Enzo Errichetti
Department of Experimental and Clinical
Medicine
Institute of Dermatology
University of Udine, Italy

Luca Feci
Department of Medical Science
Surgery and Neuroscience
Section of Dermatology
University of Siena, Italy

Salvatore Ferraro
Dermatology Clinic
University of Catania, Italy

Giorgio Filosa
Dermatology Unit "Carlo Urbani" Hospital
Jesi, Italy

Michele Fimiani
Department of Medical Science
Surgery and Neuroscience
Section of Dermatology
University of Siena, Italy

Begoña García-García
Department of Dermatology
Hospital Universitario Central de Asturias
Oviedo, Asturias, Spain

Celia Gómez de Castro
Department of Dermatology
Hospital Universitario Central de Asturias
Oviedo, Asturias, Spain

Francesco Lacarrubba
Dermatology Clinic
University of Catania, Italy

Aimilios Lallas
First Department of Dermatology
Aristotle University
Thessaloniki, Greece

Filomena Mandato
Department of Medical Science
Surgery and Neuroscience
Section of Dermatology
University of Siena, Italy

Giuseppe Micali
Dermatology Clinic
University of Catania, Italy

Sara Mohy
Misr University for Science and Technology
Giza, Egypt

Hoda Monieb
Ain Shams University
Cairo Egypt

Elvira Moscarella
Skin Cancer Unit
Arcispedale S.Maria Nuova
Reggio Emilia, Italy

Maria Letizia Musumeci
Dermatology Clinic
University of Catania, Italy

Niccolò Nami
Department of Medical Science
Surgery and Neuroscience
Section of Dermatology
University of Siena, Italy

Maria Rita Nasca
Dermatology Clinic
University of Catania, Italy

Maria Concetta Potenza
Dermatology Unit, Polo Pontino
University of Rome "Sapienza"
Rome, Italy

Ilaria Proietti
Dermatology Unit, Polo Pontino
University of Rome "Sapienza"
Rome, Italy

Paolo Rosina
Department of Medicine
Section of Dermatology and Venereology
University of Verona, Italy

Pietro Rubegni
Department of Medical Science
Surgery and Neuroscience
Section of Dermatology
University of Siena, Italy

Cecilia Santagati
Dermatology Clinic
University of Catania, Italy

Wael Saudi
Misr University for Science and Technology
Cairo, Egypt

Robert A. Schwartz
Department of Dermatology and Pathology
Rutgers University Medical School
Newark, New Jersey, USA

Michael D. Southall
Johnson & Johnson Skin Research Center
CPPW
Johnson & Johnson Consumer Companies Inc.
Skillman, New Jersey, USA

Leonardo Spagnol Abraham
Department of Dermatology
Universidade de Brasília, Brasília, Brazil

Contributors

Giuseppe Stinco
Department of Experimental and Clinical Medicine
Institute of Dermatology
University of Udine, Italy

Aurora Tedeschi
Dermatology Clinic
University of Catania, Italy

Linda Tognetti
Department of Medical Science
Surgery and Neuroscience
Section of Dermatology
University of Siena, Italy

Antonella Tosti
Department of Dermatology and Cutaneous Surgery
University of Miami Miller School of Medicine
Miami, Florida, USA

Felipe Valdes Pineda
Department of Dermatology
Hospital Universitario Central de Asturias
Oviedo, Asturias, Spain

Francisco Vazquez Lopez
Department of Dermatology
Hospital Universitario Central de Asturias
Oviedo, Asturias, Spain

Anna Elisa Verzì
Dermatology Clinic
University of Catania, Italy

Dennis P. West
Department of Dermatology
Feinberg School of Medicine
Northwestern University
Chicago, Illinois, USA

Pedro Zaballos Diego
Dermatology Department
Hospital de Sant Pau i Santa Tecla
Spain

1 Equipment for dermatoscopy/videodermatoscopy

Pietro Rubegni, Niccolò Nami, Luca Feci, Marco Burroni, Linda Tognetti, and Michele Fimiani

DERMATOSCOPY

The optical dermatoscope is an instrument containing a light source that enables skin structures invisible to the naked eye to be seen. A medium such as ultrasound gel or vaseline oil is applied to the skin to make the stratum corneum transparent (epiluminescence technique), and the dermatoscope lens is placed against the skin surface. The instrument makes it possible to observe a vast new range of dermatological signs. A limitation of the handheld dermatoscope is represented by maximum ×10 magnification. In addition, many devices do not allow image storage, although new models can be connected to photocameras or smartphones for storage and post-processing.

Dermatoscopy is currently used in routine dermatology. The various specialist courses held in recent years have led to the definition of new methods for improving the diagnosis of neoplastic and other skin disorders.

VIDEODERMATOSCOPY

ANALOG VIDEODERMATOSCOPY

Between 1980 and 1990, advances in video technology led to the development of instruments that displayed dermatoscopic images on a screen.[1] The first videodermatoscopes had a telecamera with video resolution connected to an optical dermatoscope and a television screen with video recorders to record examinations. They suffered from low quality due to the low resolution of the first video cameras and cumbersome documentation and data-saving procedures. Maximum television resolution is 768 × 576 pixel for the European PAL Broadcast system and less for the US National Television Systems Committee (NTSC) where pixel is the basic image unit; analog video recorders of the 1980s often had less than 400 horizontal lines. Low quality and technical limitations prevented the widespread use of videodermatoscopy.[2]

DIGITAL VIDEODERMATOSCOPY

Between 1990 and 2000, computerized instruments for digitizing images from telecameras connected to videodermatoscopes became common. Digital dermatoscopic images can be obtained by conversion from video-telecameras connected to digital cards or by use of high-resolution digital telecameras or digital cameras coupled with special dermatoscopy adaptors. Computerized systems proved more practical for managing examinations because they offered the possibility of saving personal and private data of patients together with digital images of pigmented skin lesions (Figure 1.1).[2-3]

In the case of video-telecameras, the signal acquisition peripheral required a charge coupled device (3CCD) or sensor for the red, green, and blue bands, to keep image quality high during sampling.[1,4] Digital telecameras have better quality for the equivalent video characteristics because they do not require any conversion. They can have a USB (usually amateur grade) or Firewire (professional grade faster and better quality) interface. Much higher resolution is possible with digital telecameras than with analog video telecameras, and this has clear diagnostic advantages, as digital dermatoscopy systems of this type can reach 1280 × 1024 pixel with images observed *in vivo* at 15–25 photograms per second on computer screens (Figure 1.2). Digital cameras provide exceptionally high resolutions (up to 3000 × 2000 are common) but

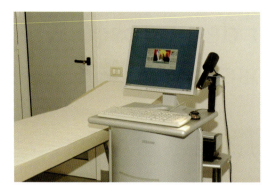

FIGURE 1.1 Digital videodermatoscope.

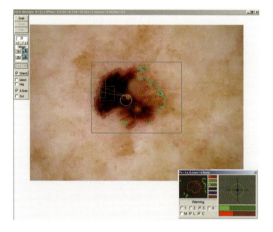

FIGURE 1.2 "Real-time" digital dermatoscopy analyzer.

have the disadvantage of not providing full-resolution images *in vivo* but only after the images have been saved.

The two types of digital instruments are therefore designed for different users. Clinicians who use video or digital telecameras (usually specialist centers) perform many examinations to diagnose melanoma or inflammatory skin diseases and observe many lesions by digital technology. Digital cameras are largely used to document lesions first observed by traditional dermatoscopy.[5]

It is commonly thought that a higher number of pixels implies better quality images; this is untrue, even if *resolution* is the imaging system's ability to reproduce details. Image quality is determinant for early diagnosis of melanoma and depends on factors such as the optical system of the instrument, illumination, type of instrument, and resolution.[6] Digital dermatoscopy images generally have between 768×576 and 1600×1200 pixel; lower resolution compromises diagnosis and higher resolution is unnecessary (Figure 1.3). The definition of magnification is only valid for integrated instruments with the same screens. *Field of view* is a preferable parameter. Dermatoscopy optical systems generally enable a horizontal field of view between 2 mm and 3 cm to be viewed. Overall magnification M of digital dermatoscopes is calculated as the ratio of screen diagonal D to field of view diagonal d: $M = D/d$.

Illumination must be homogeneous and sufficiently strong, while incident intensity should be modified by the lens diaphragm rather than

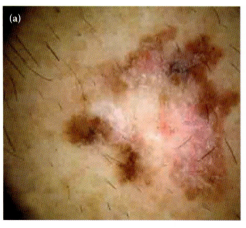 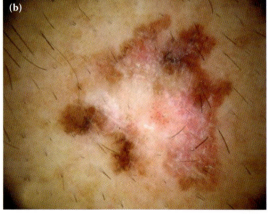

FIGURE 1.3 (a) Dermatoscopic image at 512×384 pixel resolution (42.8 KB). (b) The same image at 1024×768 pixel resolution (326 KB).

by varying electrical potential, to keep the color of the study area constant. Reddish or saturated images result from low-quality equipment or failure to balance white during chromatic calibration.

On the basis of the observation that in adult patients benign lesions remain stable whereas melanoma tends to grow and change over time, digital follow-up of melanocytic lesions has been proposed as a strategy to recognize melanoma. Stratification of the risk of developing melanoma is of great importance to establish the best strategies and follow-up methods. The intervals between successive dermatoscopy examinations vary. Most frequently the first checkup is performed 3 months after initial examination; further follow-up is performed every 12 months. Short-term follow-up is oriented toward assessment of single melanocytic lesions, while medium (every 6 months) and long-term (every 12 months) follow-up is focused on monitoring of multiple lesions. The lesions selected for short-term follow-up usually fall into two categories: moderately atypical lesions without a history of change and mildly atypical nevi with a history of change. Long-term follow-up is used for the surveillance of patients with atypical mole syndrome or high nevi count, among other risk factors. Short-term follow-up (after 3 months) may be the only way to recognize early melanoma.[7–8]

CONTACT, NONCONTACT, AND POLARIZED DERMATOSCOPY

Today there are many types of dermatoscopes. Contact incident-light dermatoscopes use a glass window placed in contact with the skin, illuminated at an angle of about 30–45 degrees so as to eliminate direct reflection, and a magnifying lens system.[9] A liquid fills the space between the skin and the glass, rendering the skin translucent and revealing subcutaneous patterns invisible to the naked eye.[9–11]

Two polarizing filters can be added to this simple optical system, one before the telecamera sensor and one on the light source, to eliminate light reflected by cross-polarization. Light reflected from the skin surface maintaining the polarization of the light source is eliminated by the polarizer in front of the sensor; this enables skin patterns to be observed to a greater depth.

Polarization makes it possible to dispense with the glass window in contact with the skin. This has the advantage of avoiding transmission of infections and ischemia caused by pressure of the window on the skin.[9]

DATA STORAGE

Digital telecameras and photocameras are now used in all medical centers, especially dermatology clinics, to acquire skin images.[12–13] Initially these instruments were not used routinely by enthusiasts, but soon the need emerged to develop software to store the data acquired. Such software enables images to be saved and stored in clinical records together with personal, confidential, and multimedia data.[14] Some examples for dermatologists are Imagestore for Healthcare, Mirror Software, and Dermo-Image (Table 1.1). Only Dermo-Image (Figure 1.4) and Imagestore for Healthcare include a preset, updatable index of dermatological disorders ready to implement.[14] The latter enables overlay of multiple images and fade between them using the *compare* feature and includes retrieval of digital images by diagnosis, treatment, and anatomical site. Mirror Software was developed specifically for medical professionals; the basic management functions of storing, retrieving, viewing, and printing images were all designed with the workflow of a medical practice in mind. The loop tool allows practitioners to critically examine skin features to target problem areas. Images can be transferred to other programs like Microsoft Word and PowerPoint. The software includes classification by pathology, patient, or examination and an advanced image retrieval system based on personalized criteria. Imagestore for Healthcare, Mirror, and Dermo-Image have these features and also enable comparison of two or more digital images. This function is useful for assessing results of treatment and evolution of lesions.[15]

SOFTWARE FOR OBJECTIVE ASSESSMENT AND ASSISTED DIAGNOSIS

The idea of a computer being able to perform a medical diagnosis is not new, with the theoretical foundations of the modern Medical

TABLE 1.1
Selected commercially available database software for dermatological digital image management

Software/Contact	Specifically for Dermatology (Preset Updatable Index and Tags)	Specific Tags for Image Retrieval	Image Modification tool	Confidentiality with Username and Password Protection	Network Compatible with Image Sharing via the Net	History Import Option	Cost
Mirror Software www.canfieldsci.com/Imaging_Products_Imaging.asp	No	Yes	Only in the $2500 or over version	Yes	Yes	No	$825 ($2500 with DPS tools)
Imagestore for Healthcare www.ttlsoftware.com	Yes	Yes	Yes	Securely access images from any Internet-connected PC	Yes	No	Not available
Dermo-Image www.dermoimage.com	Yes	Yes	Yes	Powerful and flexible permission system	Yes	Yes	$900

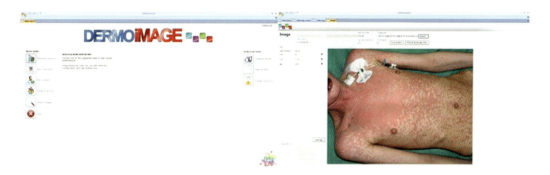

FIGURE 1.4 Dermo-Image software for image storage (Ergon srl, Siena, Italy; dermoimage@ergonsrl.it).

Diagnosis Decision Support having been laid as early as the 1950s. Calculators with memory can keep track of more things and perform calculations faster than the brightest humans. However, in many cases the problem has a solution that can be found quickly using common sense. In such case, the brute-force method machines required could never compete with humans. This is the key to the proper use of any computation machine, above all in the medical setting. When common sense does not provide a quick solution, a machine can facilitate the exploration of the possible reasons for a patient's illness. A machine can keep track of more findings, possible conclusions, and disease and test parameters than most clinicians. If common sense could be partnered with machines, the result would be better than either could provide alone. If together they can improve the accuracy, speed, and efficiency of diagnosis, the combination of man and machine in medicine provides value.

In the field of dermatology, many research groups have worked on image processing and numerical assessment of image features for diagnostic purposes in the last few years (Table 1.2). The process generally consists of detecting the borders of the skin area to assess, identifying the object(s) to examine, and evaluating a number of variables to differentiate various diagnostic situations (Figure 1.5). Many studies have been concerned with objective computerized analysis of digital images acquired by dermatoscopy.[16–18] In the case of pigmented skin lesions, this has involved identification of variables such as circularity, maximum diameter, symmetry, and internal clusters of color, for objective evaluation of all possible types.[17] The new path taken by researchers envisages definition of new, unambiguous, reproducible variables. Objective evaluation also offers the opportunity of using assisted diagnosis systems to provide diagnostic suggestions.[19–20] On the basis of morpho-chromatic characteristics of lesions, it is possible to build a classifier that can evaluate the statistical probability of malignancy with the aid of a special thesaurus.

These instruments have also been used in trichology and aesthetics with interesting results. Sensitive tools have been developed to monitor hair loss and treatment responses. The Trichoscan was launched as a method combining epiluminescence microscopy with automatic digital image analysis.[21]

CONCLUSIONS

The continuing evolution of digital imaging has led to the obsolescence of costly video equipment and the introduction of new digital cameras and telecameras that offer greater chromatic and spatial quality. Through this technology, dermatologists are discovering new horizons for research, teaching, and health care. In particular, using diagnostic melanoma tools as an adjunct to the clinical examination, dermatologists have the opportunity to increase both their sensitivity and specificity for melanoma detection.[22–24]

TABLE 1.2
Instruments for digital dermatoscopy analysis

Instrument	Website (www.)	Light Source	Magnification	Camera	Board	Software
DB-Mips	skinlesions.net	Halogen, 3200°K, 150 W	×16–25, global	3CCD, 750 lines	768 × 576 lines, RBG sync, 16M colors	Medical records processing, 2 statistical classifiers (neural network, similarity)
Molemax II	derma.co.at	Circular polarized	×30 fixed	1CCD	Not reported	Medical record db image processing, statistical classifier (diagnostic algorithms)
Videocap	dsmedigroup.it	Halogen, 3200°K, 150 W	×10, ×25, ×50, ×100, ×200, ×400, ×500, ×700	1CCD	PCI multi-input, 16M colors	Medical records, db images, measurements
Dermogenius	dermogenious.com	Not reported	Fixed	1CCD or 3CCD	Not reported	Medical records processing, statistical classifier (diagnostic algorithms)
Microderm	visiomed.de	Not reported	Variable but not reported	3CCD	Not reported	Medical records processing, statistical classifier (neural network)
Solarscan	polartechnics.com.av	Halogen	×10	1CCD or 3CCD	Not reported	Medical record processing, statistical classifier

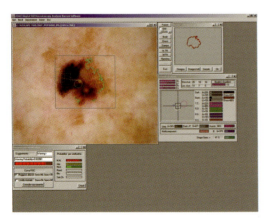

FIGURE 1.5 Images can be stored and analyzed (DB-Mips System; Biomips srl, Siena, Italy) with a computerized instrument providing a visual database and objective evaluations of pigmented skin lesions.

REFERENCES

1. Gutenev A, Skladnev VN, Varvel D. Acquisition-time image quality control in digital dermatoscopy of skin lesions. *Comput Med Imaging Graph*. 2001;25:495–99.
2. Schindewolf T, Schiffner R, Stolz W, et al. Evaluation of different image acquisition techniques for a computer vision system in the diagnosis of malignant melanoma. *J Am Acad Dermatol*. 1994;31(1):33–41.
3. Elbaum M. Computer-aided melanoma diagnosis. *Dermatol Clin*. 2002;20(4):735–47.
4. Sheeler I, Koczan P, Wallage W, de Lusignan S. Low-cost three-channel video for assessment of the clinical consultation. *Inform Prim Care*. 2007;15(1):25-31.
5. Ratner D, Thomas CO, Bickers D. The uses of digital photography in dermatology. *J Am Acad Dermatol*. 1999;41:749–56.

6. Levy JL, Trelles MA, Levy A, Besson R. Photography in dermatology: Comparison between slides and digital imaging. *J Cosmet Dermatol*. 2003;2:131–34.
7. Lallas A, Apalla Z, Chaidemenos G. New trends in dermoscopy to minimize the risk of missing melanoma. *J Skin Cancer*. 2012;2012:820474.
8. Salerni G, Carrera C, Lovatto L, et al. Characterization of 1152 lesions excised over 10 years using total-body photography and digital dermatoscopy in the surveillance of patients at high risk for melanoma. *J Am Acad Dermatol*. 2012;67:836–45.
9. Benvenuto-Andrade C, Dusza SW, Agero AL, et al. Differences between polarized light dermoscopy and immersion contact dermoscopy for the evaluation of skin lesions. *Arch Dermatol*. 2007;143(3):329–38.
10. Wang SQ, Dusza SW, Scope A, et al. Differences in dermoscopic images from non-polarized dermoscope and polarized dermoscope influence the diagnostic accuracy and confidence level: a pilot study. *Dermatol Surg*. 2008;34(10):1389–95.
11. Pan Y, Gareau DS, Scope A, et al. Polarized and nonpolarized dermoscopy: The explanation for the observed differences. *Arch Dermatol*. 2008;144(6):828–29.
12. Scheinfeld NS, Flanigan K, Moshiyakhov M, Weinberg JM. Trends in the use of cameras and computer technology among dermatologists in New York City 2001–2002. *Dermatol Surg*. 2003;29:822–25.
13. Graschew G, Roelofs TA, Rakowsky S, et al. New trends in the virtualization of hospitals-tools for global e-Health. *Stud Health Technol Inform*. 2006;121:168–75.
14. Starr JC. Integrating digital image management software for improved patient care and optimal practice management. *Dermatol Surg*. 2006;32:834–40.
15. Rubegni P, Nami N, Tataranno D, Fimiani M. Gestione delle immagini digitali. Un software dedicato per la gestione dell'archivio elettronico. *Hitechdermo*. 2008;3(3):43–49.
16. Pressley ZM, Foster JK, Kolm P, et al. Digital image analysis: a reliable tool in the quantitative evaluation of cutaneous lesions and beyond. *Arch Dermatol*. 2007;143(10):1331–33.
17. Rubegni P, Burroni M, Andreassi A, Fimiani M. The role of dermoscopy and digital dermoscopy analysis in the diagnosis of pigmented skin lesions. *Arch Dermatol*. 2005;141:1444–46.
18. Rubegni P, Burroni M, Sbano P, Andreassi L. Digital dermoscopy analysis and internet-based program for discrimination of pigmented skin lesion dermoscopic images. *Br J Dermatol*. 2005;152(2):395–96.
19. Perrinaud A, Gaide O, French LE, et al. Can automated dermoscopy image analysis instruments provide added benefit for the dermatologist? A study comparing the results of three systems. *Br J Dermatol*. 2007;157(5):926–33.
20. Piccolo D, Ferrari A, Peris K, et al. Dermoscopic diagnosis by a trained clinician vs. a clinician with minimal dermoscopy training vs. computer-aided diagnosis of 341 pigmented skin lesions: A comparative study. *Br J Dermatol*. 2002;147(3):481–86.
21. Hoffmann R, Van Neste D. Recent findings with computerized methods for scalp hair growth measurements. *J Investig Dermatol Symp Proc*. 2005;10(3):285–88.
22. Rubegni P, Cevenini G, Nami N, et al. Dermoscopy and digital dermoscopy analysis of palmoplantar "equivocal" pigmented skin lesions in Caucasians. *Dermatology*. 2012;225:248–55.
23. Kardynal A, Olszewska M. Modern non-invasive diagnostic techniques in the detection of early cutaneous melanoma. *J Dermatol Case Rep*. 2014;8(1):1–8.
24. Wassef C, Rao BK. Uses of non-invasive imaging in the diagnosis of skin cancer: An overview of the currently available modalities. *Int J Dermatol*. 2013;52(12):1481–89.

2 Parasitoses
Scabies

Giuseppe Micali, Francesco Lacarrubba, and Robert A. Schwartz

DEFINITION

Scabies is a common ectoparasitosis caused by the mite *Sarcoptes scabiei hominis*.[1]

EPIDEMIOLOGY/ETIOPATHOGENESIS

Scabies is endemic worldwide, particularly in impoverished communities; epidemics can occur during famine and war. The global estimated prevalence is about 300 million cases. Scabies is not affected by gender or race. In industrialized nations, it is usually observed in sporadic individual cases and institutional outbreaks (hospitals, nursing homes, prisons, and elementary schools). Risk factors include poverty, poor nutrition, homelessness, dementia, and poor hygiene.[2,3] Transmission is by direct skin-to-skin contact through close personal contact, sexual or otherwise, or, less frequently, indirectly via fomite transmission (clothing, bedsheets, etc).

Adult females of the mite are between 0.3 and 0.5 mm long; males are smaller, reaching 0.21–0.29 mm,[4–5] with four pairs of legs. The mites can crawl up to 2.5 cm per minute on warm skin and live approximately 30 days.[6,7] Females dig tunnel-like burrows in the stratum corneum and lay approximately 2–3 eggs daily. An infested host contains approximately 10–15 adult female mites on his or her body at any given time. However, in crusted or Norwegian scabies, which is found most commonly in HIV (human immunodeficiency virus) patients, the elderly, or other immunosuppressed individuals, the mite burden can total over 1 million. *S. scabiei* can survive outside of the host for up to 24–36 hours.[8–9]

CLINICAL PRESENTATION/DIAGNOSIS

The pathognomonic sign of scabies is the burrow (Figure 2.1), which represents the tunnel that a female mite excavates while laying eggs. It is a white serpiginous line ranging from 1–10 mm in length typically located on the interdigital spaces of the hand, the flexure surface of the wrist, elbows, genitalia, axillae, umbilicus, belt line, elbows, nipples, buttocks, and penile shaft. Nocturnal pruritus and erythematous papules also form the basis of diagnosis, and result from a delayed type IV hypersensitivity reaction to the mite, its saliva, eggs, or excrement (scybala). Even after successful treatment, pruritus and lesions can persist for 2–4 weeks ("post-scabietic pruritus").[10–11] Secondary bacterial infection commonly occurs in the lesions, particularly in the hands and feet of young children, and should be treated first.

The differential diagnosis of scabies is extensive and includes atopic dermatitis, neurodermatitis, animal scabies (whose mites cannot complete the life cycle on human hosts because they cannot burrow), papular urticaria, folliculitis, dermatitis herpetiformis, prurigo nodularis, and bites from mosquitoes, fleas, bedbugs, chiggers, or other mites.[12–18]

The standard technique for the diagnosis of scabies consists of identification of the mite, eggs, or feces by microscopic examination of scales obtained by skin scraping. Scrapings should preferably be from a fresh, non-excoriated burrow in the interdigital areas of the hand. Often repeated scrapings are needed because the sensitivity is quite low. Skin scraping may be too discomforting and may cause fear, especially in younger patients. As the results generally depend on the scraped areas, repeated tests are

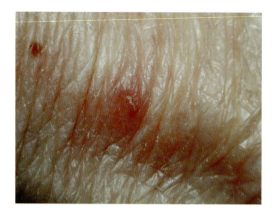

FIGURE 2.1 The burrow, a pathognomonic sign of scabies.

sometimes necessary for a conclusive diagnosis. For these reasons, scraping is not well accepted by patients, who may not cooperate or may even decline the examination. Follow-up tests, useful to assess recovery from therapy or to rule out persisting pruritus due to use of irritant topical agents, are troublesome, and patients may refuse further scraping, considering it useless "torture." Moreover, handling and processing scrapings rapidly and effectively in the office is not always straightforward.[19–20]

DERMATOSCOPY/VIDEODERMATOSCOPY FEATURES

In 1992 Kreusch[21] suggested the use of epiluminescence microscopy in diagnosing scabies, as this technique allows the inspection of the skin surface down to the superficial dermis. The first study was performed by Argenziano and colleagues five years later;[22] the authors, using the epiluminescence microscopy technique at ×40 magnification, detected in 93% of 70 patients affected by scabies a repetitive finding consisting of a small, dark brown triangular structure located at the end of a subtle linear segment; together, both structures resembled a jet with contrail.[22–23] On microscopic examination, the jet-shaped triangular structure corresponded to the pigmented anterior part of the mite (mouth parts and two anterior pairs of legs); the contrail-shaped segment was thought to be the burrow of the mite along with its eggs and fecal pellets.[22–23]

In 2000 a comparative study[24] of scraping versus high-magnification videodermatoscopy (VD) was performed in 38 patients suspected of being infested with scabies (age 1 month to 81 years). Two independent operators performed both scraping and VD examinations in each patient; exchange of information was not allowed. The use of VD allowed a detailed inspection of the skin with rapid identification of burrows, mites, feces, and eggs in 16 of 38 patients. In most cases, it was possible to observe the mites moving inside the burrows. Microscopic examination of the scales obtained by skin scraping gave similar results. Interestingly, two cases were positive only by scraping, and this fact was probably due to impetiginization that hampered VD examination (Figure 2.2); conversely, two other cases, characterized by minimal lesions, were found positive only at VD (Figure 2.3).

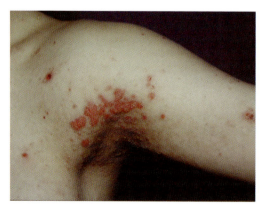

FIGURE 2.2 A case of super-infected scabies in which VD examination may be hampered and may give a false negative result.

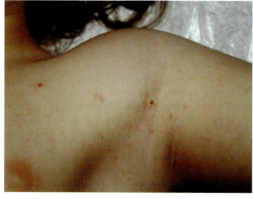

FIGURE 2.3 A case of scabies with minimal lesions, in which traditional skin scraping examination may give a false negative result.

A larger study was performed in children.[19] One hundred young patients (43 male, 57 female; age range 1 month to 16 years) suspected to be affected by scabies were enrolled in the study. Patient examination was first performed using ×100 magnification, and suspicious lesions (i.e., burrows) were analyzed at higher magnification (up to ×600). Diagnosis of scabies was established in 62 of 100 patients and was based on identification of mite migration and identification of eggs and feces. None of the 38 negative patients showed signs of infestation at a 2-week follow-up examination, ruling out the possibility of "false negative" results. The study showed that high magnification VD is very effective and sensitive, especially in cases with nonspecific clinical features, allowing clear detection of some details (e.g., mites in migration, eggs, and feces) usually not appreciable at lower magnifications.[19]

A study comparing the diagnosis of scabies using a pocket handheld dermatoscope allowing ×10 magnification with traditional skin scraping in 238 patients has shown that dermatoscopy achieves comparable high-diagnostic sensitivity values as scraping (91% vs. 90%, respectively). Under ×10 magnification, after paraffin oil application on the glass plate of the dermatoscope, *S. scabiei* appears as a characteristic triangular shape resembling a circumflex accent (e.g., in French letter 'ô'), which corresponds to the head and front legs of the mite.[25] The effectiveness of dermatoscopy both at low and high magnification in diagnosing scabies has been confirmed by several other studies.[20,26–31]

Dermatoscopy affords several advantages compared to traditional skin scraping. First, it is not invasive and it is well accepted by patients, especially by children and those more sensitive patients who may have had repeated negative results from skin scraping, as it does not cause physical or psychological discomfort. It is easy and quick to perform, allowing inspection of the entire skin surface usually within a few minutes, significantly less time-consuming than *ex vivo* microscopic examination.[19,23] It is useful for nontraumatic screening of family members who might decline skin scraping because they are asymptomatic. Moreover, because it is noninvasive, this technique minimizes the risk of accidental infections from blood-transmissible agents such as Human Immunodeficiency Virus (HIV) or Hepatitis C Virus (HCV). Finally, dermatoscopy has demonstrated to be useful in diagnosing scabies through the technique of teledermatology. In one study this approach, which involves sharing digital pictures by capturing dermatoscopic images at the remote site and reviewing them later at the host site, appeared to be a relatively cost-effective means of providing this service from a distance when on-site dermatology services are absent.[32]

An important issue to address is which magnification gives the best performance, considering that most systems are equipped with lenses up to ×200. The use of VD, whenever possible, is recommended, as it allows a detailed inspection of the skin with rapid and clear detection of the diagnostic features of scabies, such as burrows at magnifications ranging ×40 to ×100, and mites, eggs, or feces at higher magnifications (up to ×600) (Figures 2.4–2.7). Using these magnifications, false negative results are rare and there is no chance of false positive results, as the images obtained are unequivocal: the roundish translucent body of the mite (invisible at low magnifications) is clearly visible, and it is always possible to visualize the other anatomical structures of the mite, such as its legs (anterior and posterior) and rostrum; in most cases, it is also possible to detect the mite moving inside the burrows.[24,26] The use of oil and slides that are messy and time-consuming is unnecessary at high magnification, because they do not enhance diagnostic capability.

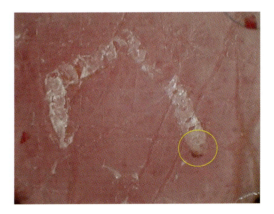

FIGURE 2.4 VD of a burrow: the roundish body of *Sarcoptes scabiei* may be observed at one end (circle) (×100).

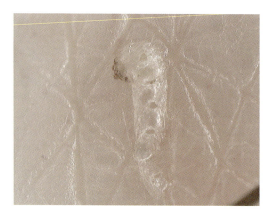

FIGURE 2.5 VD of a burrow: *Sarcoptes scabiei* is clearly visible (×200).

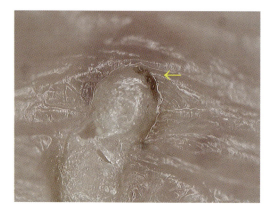

FIGURE 2.6 VD of *Sarcoptes scabiei:* the roundish body is translucent, while the anterior part of the mite (head and anterior legs) is pigmented (arrow) (×500).

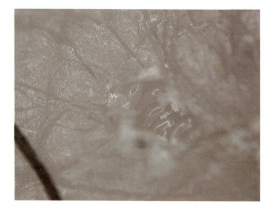

FIGURE 2.7 VD of eggs (ovular and translucent) and feces (roundish and white) of *Sarcoptes scabiei* (×500).

A limitation of the use of VD devices is their high cost. However, low-cost videomicroscopes (VMs) allowing magnification up to ×1000 (cost is about $30) are available for nonmedical use in entomology, botany, and/or microelectronics. In a recent study of 20 patients with presumed scabies infestation, two nonmedical videomicroscopes have been compared to a medically marketed videodermatoscope.[33] At the end of the study, the VMs allowed for a definitive scabies diagnosis, as did the VD, enabling an adequate and optimal visualization of the typical signs. The impact of inexpensive VMs appears to be significant and cost-effective, both in institutional settings such as hospitals, nursing homes, long-term care facilities, and prisons, and in underdeveloped countries experiencing endemic outbreaks, where noninvasive techniques and low costs are essential.[33]

In conclusion, the use of noninvasive technique may undoubtedly enhance the diagnosis of scabies. However, low-magnification devices (×10–×40) may have some limitations. One is that they do not always allow, especially to inexperienced operators, a clear differentiation between the "circumflex accent" (or the "jet-shaped" structure) and minor excoriations and/or splinters (that may frequently occur in scabies due to repeated scratching). In addition, low magnifications do not allow eggs and feces visualization that may often be the only diagnostic clues. Another limitation is that mite viability cannot be assessed at these magnifications, so that posttherapeutic monitoring cannot be performed. Finally, the use of handheld dermatoscopy may be troublesome on hairy body areas where a clear visualization of the skin may be hampered. In addition, its use in or around the genital region may cause embarrassment because of close contact between the dermatoscopist's head and the patient's skin surface.[25] In conclusion, because of the possible risk of false negative and/or false positive results, the use of handheld dermatoscopy might be reserved for those cases in which no VD facilities are available or for a preliminary screening of suspect lesions before skin scraping.

The importance of the use of high magnifications may be better understood by viewing the same lesion at different magnifications (Figures 2.8–2.9).

Parasitoses

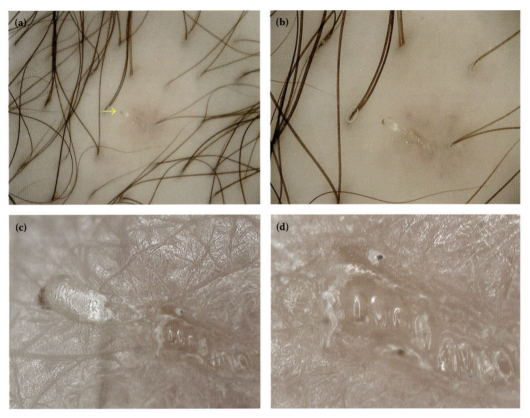

FIGURE 2.8 (a) Low-magnification VD (×20) of a burrow: the circumflex accent, which corresponds to the head and front legs of the mite structure, may be observed (arrow). (b) ×40 magnification VD of the same burrow: the jet with contrail structure is more evident. (c) ×400 magnification VD of the same burrow: both the mite (on the left) and the eggs (on the right) are clearly evident. (d) Eggs at ×600 magnification.

Finally, when using the dermatoscope or the videodermatoscope in a patient affected by scabies, the possibility of indirect contamination through the instrument might be considered, as mites survive in the environment for up to 36 hours; thus, accurate cleaning and disinfection of the device after each examination is recommended.[25]

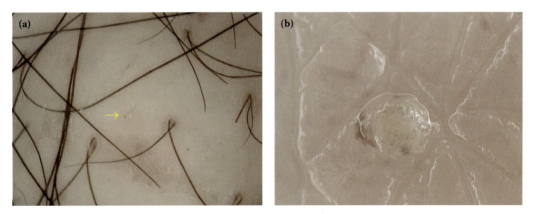

FIGURE 2.9 *Sarcoptes scabiei* out of the burrow. (a) At low-magnification VD the circumflex accent (arrow) is hardly visible (×20). (b) The same mite at higher magnification is easily recognizable (×500).

REFERENCES

1. Hengge UR, Currie BJ, Jager G, et al. Scabies: A ubiquitous neglected skin disease. *Lancet Infect Dis*. 2006;6:769–79.
2. Badiaga S, Menard A, Tissot Dupont H, et al. Prevalence of skin infections in sheltered homeless. *Eur J Dermatol*. 2005;15:382–86.
3. Tsutsumi M, Nishiura H, Kobayashi T. Dementia-specific risks of scabies: Retrospective epidemiologic analysis of an unveiled nosocomial outbreak in Japan from 1989–90. *BMC Infect Dis*. 2005;5:85.
4. Burgess I. Sarcoptes scabiei and scabies. *Adv Parasitol*. 1994;33:235–92.
5. Walton SF, Currie BJ. Problems in diagnosing scabies, a global disease in human and animal populations. *Clin Microbiol Rev*. 2007;20:268–79.
6. Sterling GB, Janniger CK, Kihiczak G, et al. Scabies. *Am Fam Physician*. 1992;46:1237–41.
7. Molinaro MJ, Schwartz RA, Janniger CK. Scabies. *Cutis*. 1995;56:317–21.
8. Arlian LG, Runyan RA, Achar S, Estes SA. Survival and infectivity of *Sarcoptes scabiei var. canis* and *var. hominis*. *J Am Acad Dermatol*. 1984;11:210–15.
9. Heukelbach J, Feldmeier H. Scabies. *Lancet*. 2006;367:1767–74.
10. Janniger CK, Micali G, Hengge U, et al. Scabies. *eMedicine Pediatrics* [journal serial online]. 2008. Available at http://author.emedicine.com/ped/topic2047.htm.
11. Chosidow O. Scabies and pediculosis. *Lancet*. 2000;355:819–26.
12. Stibich AS, Schwartz RA. Papular urticaria. *Cutis*. 2001;68:89–91.
13. Steen CJ, Carbonaro PA, Schwartz RA. Arthropods in dermatology. *J Am Acad Dermatol*. 2004;50:819–42, quiz 42-4.
14. Thomas I, Kihiczak GG, Schwartz RA. Bedbug bites: A review. *Int J Dermatol*. 2004;43:430–33.
15. Nutanson I, Steen C, Schwartz RA. Pediculosis corporis: An ancient itch. *Acta Dermatovenerol Croat*. 2007;15:33–38.
16. Vaidya DC, Schwartz RA. Prurigo nodularis: A benign dermatosis derived from a persistent pruritus. *Acta Dermatovenerol Croat*. 2008;16:38–44.
17. Schwartz RA. Papular Urticaria. Medscape Reference. Updated April 15, 2014. Available at: http://emedicine.medscape.com/article/ 1051461-overview.
18. Schwartz RA. Bedbug Bites. Medscape Reference. Updated May 11, 2015. Available at: http://emedicine.medscape.com/article/ 1088931-overview.
19. Lacarrubba F, Musumeci ML, Caltabiano R, et al. High-magnification videodermatoscopy: A new noninvasive diagnostic tool for scabies in children. *Ped Dermatol*. 2001;18:439–41.
20. Neynaber S, Wolff H. Diagnosis of scabies with dermoscopy. *CMAJ*. 2008;178:1540–41.
21. Kreusch J. Incident light microscopy: Reflection on microscopy of the living skin. *Int J Dermatol*. 1992;31:618–20.
22. Argenziano G, Fabbrocini G, Delfino M. Epiluminescence microscopy. A new approach to *in vivo* detection of Sarcoptes scabiei. *Arch Dermatol*. 1997;133:751–53.
23. Zalaudek I, Giacomel J, Cabo H, et al. Entodermoscopy: A new tool for diagnosing skin infections and infestations. *Dermatology*. 2008;216:14–23.
24. Micali G, Lacarrubba F, Lo Guzzo G. Scraping versus videodermatoscopy for the diagnosis of scabies: A comparative study (Letter). *Acta Derm Venereol*. 2000;79:396.
25. Dupuy A, Dehen L, Bourrat E, et al. Accuracy of standard dermoscopy for diagnosing scabies. *J Am Acad Dermatol*. 2007;56:53–62.
26. Brunetti B, Vitiello A, Delfino S, Sammarco E. Findings *in vivo* of *Sarcoptes scabiei* with incident light microscopy. *Eur J Dermatol*. 1998;8:266–67.
27. Bauer J, Blum A, Sönnichsen K, et al. Nodular scabies detected by computed dermatoscopy. *Dermatology*. 2001;203(2):190–91.
28. Prins C, Stucki L, French L, et al. Dermoscopy for the *in vivo* detection of *Sarcoptes scabiei*. *Dermatology*. 2004;208:241–43.
29. Fox GN, Usatine RP. Itching and rash in a boy and his grandmother. *J Fam Pract*. 2006;55:679–84.
30. Executive Committee of Guideline for the Diagnosis, Ishii N. Guideline for the diagnosis and treatment of scabies in Japan (second edition). *J Dermatol*. 2008;35:378–93.
31. Lacarrubba F, Micali G. Videodermatoscopy and scabies. *J Pediatr*. 2013;163:1227–1227.e1.
32. Weinstock MA, Kempton SA. Case report: Teledermatology and epiluminescence microscopy for the diagnosis of scabies. *Cutis*. 2000;66:61–62.
33. Micali G, Lacarrubba F, Verzì AE, Nasca MR. Low cost equipment for diagnosis and management of endemic scabies outbreaks in underserved populations. *Clin Infect Dis*. 2015;60:327–29.

3 Parasitoses
Pediculosis

Francesco Lacarrubba, Giuseppe Micali, Alessandro Di Stefani, and Robert A. Schwartz

HEAD LICE

DEFINITION

Head lice, or pediculosis capitis, is a scalp infestation caused by *Pediculus humanus capitis* (Figure 3.1).

EPIDEMIOLOGY/ETIOPATHOGENESIS

Pediculosis capitis is a common health problem that affects about 6 to 12 million people every year in the United States.[1–4] Infestation occurs most commonly in children, with a peak incidence between 5 and 13 years of age. It is found worldwide without predilection for a particular age, sex, race, or socioeconomic class. Girls are twice as likely as boys to have head lice because of their longer hair and sharing of brushes and hair accessories.[5] Head lice are rare in African Americans due to the anatomy of their hair shaft, which is more oval, making it harder to be grasped.[6,7]

Pediculus humanus capitis is a host-specific arthropod that belongs to the order Anoplura. It measures approximately 2–3 mm in length and is grayish-white in color. It is wingless and has narrow sucking mouthparts concealed within the head, short antennae, and three pairs of clawed legs for hair grasping. The louse moves by grasping hairs and is incapable of flying or jumping. It feeds by piercing the skin of the host with its mouthparts and sucking blood every 4–6 hours. The female louse lives approximately 30 days and lays about 5–10 eggs a day on hair shafts. Eggs, also known as nits, are 0.8 mm in length and are laid within 1–2 mm of the scalp surface for warmth. The nits are firmly glued to the individual hairs by a proteinaceous matrix and are difficult to remove. Dead eggs can remain affixed to the hair shafts for as long as 6 months and can lead to a false-positive diagnosis of an active infestation, as it may be difficult to distinguish between viable and empty eggs. Head lice can survive for up to 3 days off the host, and nits for 10 days away from their host. Transmission is thought to occur through direct head-to-head contact for an extended period of time.

CLINICAL PRESENTATION/DIAGNOSIS

Pruritus of the scalp is the primary symptom of head lice, although a number of patients are asymptomatic and are considered carriers.[7] Occasionally, secondary bacterial infections resulting from scratching with an associated local retro-auricular adenopathy may be seen.

The diagnosis is established by identification of viable nits or an adult louse on the scalp (especially the occipital and postauricular areas), whose recognition can be facilitated through the use of a magnifying glass. Viable nits are tan to brown in color, and hatched nits are clear to white. Louse combs are useful tools, as they increase the chance of finding live lice fourfold over direct visual examination.[8,9]

Sometimes nits may be overlooked and nits containing vital nymphs can be difficult to differentiate from empty nits and so-called pseudonits, such as hair casts, debris of hair spray or gel, or scales from seborrheic dermatitis.[10] Hair casts may also closely resemble nits stuck to hair shafts and can be noticed by a parent, teacher, or school nurse who mistakes them for nits.[3] In contrast to nits, they are freely movable along the hair shaft.

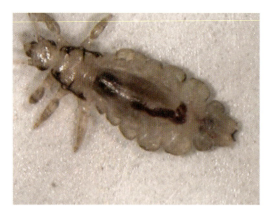

FIGURE 3.1 VD of *Pediculus humanus capitis* on a glass slide (×80).

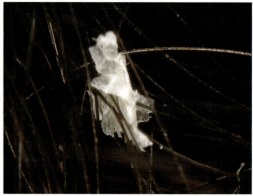

FIGURE 3.3 VD of a scale of seborrheic dermatitis (pseudo-nit) appearing as an amorphous, whitish structure (×80).

Dermatoscopy/Videodermatoscopy features

Videodermatoscopy (VD) may be used as an easy, safe, and reliable diagnostic tool in head lice infestation, rapidly confirming the diagnosis in some puzzling cases in which parasites and nits are not easily identified.[11–12] It unequivocally shows the presence of the nits fixed to the hair shaft (Figure 3.2), allowing a rapid differentiation from pseudo-nits, which appear as amorphous, whitish structures (Figure 3.3). Moreover, VD allows a more detailed identification of full versus empty nits: the first, which contain nymphs and indicate a potential active infestation, appear as ovoid, brown structures with a convex extremity (Figure 3.4a); the empty nits, which may persist after the recovery, are translucent and typically show a plane and fissured free ending (Figure 3.4b). The differentiation between vital and empty nits provides

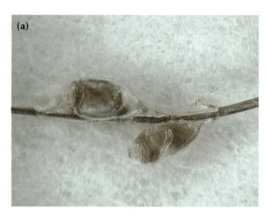

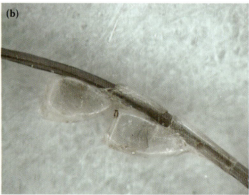

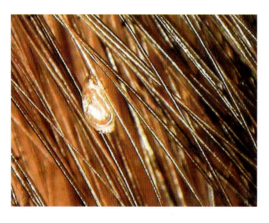

FIGURE 3.2 VD of a full nit fixed to the hair shaft (×80).

FIGURE 3.4 (a) VD of full nits, which contain nymphs, appearing as ovoid, brown structures with a convex extremity (×100). (b) VD of empty, translucent nits typically showing a plane and fissured free ending (×100).

Parasitoses

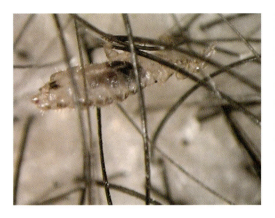

FIGURE 3.5 VD of *Pediculus humanus* "in action" in the hair shafts (×80).

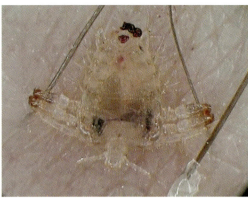

FIGURE 3.6 VD of *Phthirus pubis* firmly attached to the pubic hairs (×80).

useful information about therapeutic response. Furthermore, VD does not require hair pulling, so a large scalp area can be investigated without discomfort to the patient. With a little patience it is also possible to detect the lice. In this case VD allows an *in vivo* evaluation of the movements and physiology of lice (Figure 3.5) and may be useful to evaluate the pediculocidal activity of different topical products.[13]

Other authors have reported obtaining similar results using a contact handheld dermatoscope both *in vivo* and *ex vivo*, by nipping and placing hairs with attached nits on adhesive tape.[10, 14–15]

CRAB LICE

Definition

Crab lice, or pediculosis pubis, is a skin infestation caused by *Phthirus pubis*.

Epidemiology/Etiopathogenesis

Pubic lice infestation is a common disorder, diffused worldwide, which is spread as a sexually transmitted disease. Contamination may also occur indirectly (underwear, bedclothes). It is slightly more prevalent in men, probably due to their increased amount of coarse body hair, and is most common in subjects between 15 and 40 years old, reflecting increased sexual activity during this period.[16]

Phthirus pubis is approximately 0.8–1.2 mm, has a shorter body than head lice, and resembles microscopic crabs (Figure 3.6). The mites have serrated edges on their anterior claws allowing them increased traction and mobility on the entire body.[17] The female mites, firmly attached to pubic hairs, deliver their nits, which unfold after 7–10 days. *Phtirus pubis* is an emathophagous insect, and itching is caused by its bites.

Clinical presentation/Diagnosis

Phthirus pubis infests mainly the hair of the pubic and inguinal region (Figure 3.7), and rarely those of axillae, chest, and limbs. In children, the edges of scalp hair and eyelashes (phthiriasis palpebrarum) are the most common site of infestation because of the lack of terminal hairs on most body regions.[18] The main symptom is itching on the affected body areas, which

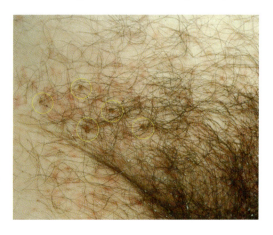

FIGURE 3.7 Crab lice (circled) of the pubic region.

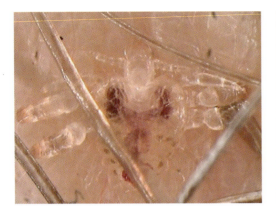

FIGURE 3.8 VD of *Phthirus pubis* (×80).

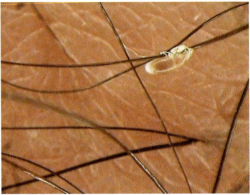

FIGURE 3.9 VD of full nit of *Phthirus pubis* (×60).

can become stronger over two or more weeks following initial infestation.

In the majority of cases the diagnosis of pubic lice is clinical and there is no need for further investigation. The identification of crab lice and their nits (0.5 mm brown-opalescent ovals) with the naked eye or a magnifying glass is diagnostic. Sometimes, nits can be misdiagnosed for white piedra or trichomycosis pubis.[19,20] When present, macula caerulea, an asymptomatic bluish-gray macula caused by a bite of the crab louse, is a characteristic finding.

Dermatoscopy/Videodermatoscopy features

Sometimes the number of living lice can be limited, and diagnosis can be aided by the use of VD to clearly show the presence of the crab lice firmly attached to the pubic hairs[11,12,21,22] (Figure 3.8). In most cases it is possible to

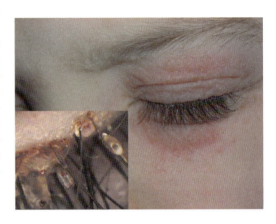

FIGURE 3.10 Phthiriasis palpebrarum. Insert: VD observation of lice and nits (×80).

recognize the parasite sucking the blood. Moreover, as observed in pediculosis capitis, VD allows a more detailed identification of full versus empty nits (Figure 3.9).

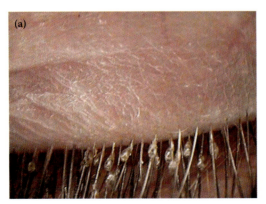
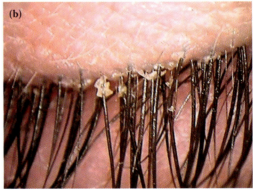

FIGURES 3.11 VD of nits (a) versus scales of atopic dermatitis (b) of the eyelashes (×30).

In the case of phthiriasis palpebrarum the lice are sometimes difficult to identify because of their semitransparency and deep burrowing in the lid margin, so the infestation may exist for a long time before being recognized[23] and may be generally misdiagnosed with atopic dermatitis or allergic conjunctivitis. In these cases VD can rapidly clarify any doubt by revealing the presence of lice and/or nits[18] (Figures 3.10–3.11).

REFERENCES

1. Chosidow O. Scabies and pediculosis. *Lancet*. 2000;355:819–26.
2. Nutanson I, Steen C, Schwartz RA. Pediculosis corporis: An ancient itch. *Acta Dermatovenerol Croat*. 2007;15:33–38.
3. Ko CJ, Elston DM. Pediculosis. *J Am Acad Dermatol*. 2004;50:1–12; quiz 3-4.
4. Nutanson I, Steen CJ, Schwartz RA, Janniger CK. Pediculosis capitis: An update. *Acta Dermatovenerol Alp Panonica Adriat*. 2008; 17:147–59.
5. Burgess I. The life of a head louse. *Nurs Times*. 2002;98:54.
6. Steen CJ, Carbonaro PA, Schwartz RA. Arthropods in dermatology. *J Am Acad Dermatol*. 2004;50:819–42, quiz 42-4.
7. Frankowski BL, Weiner LB. Head lice. *Pediatrics*. 2002;110:638–43.
8. Mumcuoglu KY, Friger M, Ioffe-Uspensky I, et al. Louse comb versus direct visual examination for the diagnosis of head louse infestations. *Pediatr Dermatol*. 2001;18:9–12.
9. De Maeseneer J, Blokland I, Willems S, et al. Wet combing versus traditional scalp inspection to detect head lice in schoolchildren: Observational study. *BMJ*. 2000;321:1187–88.
10. Di Stefani A, Hofmann-Wellenhof R, Zalaudek I. Dermoscopy for diagnosis and treatment monitoring of pediculosis capitis. *J Am Acad Dermatol*. 2006;54:909–11.
11. Micali G, Lacarrubba F. Possible applications of videodermatoscopy beyond pigmented lesions. *Int J Dermatol*. 2003;42:430–33.
12. Micali G, Lacarrubba F, Massimino D, Schwartz RA. Dermatoscopy: Alternative uses in daily clinical practice. *J Am Acad Dermatol*. 2011;64:1135–46.
13. Lacarrubba F, Nardone B, Milani M, et al. Head lice: *Ex vivo* videodermatoscopy evaluation of the pediculocidal activity of two different topical products. *G Ital Dermatol Venereol*. 2006;141:233–35.
14. Bakos RM, Bakos L. Dermoscopy for diagnosis of pediculosis capitis. *J Am Acad Dermatol*. 2007;57:727–28.
15. Zalaudek I, Giacomel J, Cabo H, et al. Entodermoscopy: A new tool for diagnosing skin infections and infestations. *Dermatology*. 2008;216:14–23.
16. Mimouni D, Ankol OE, Gdalevich M, et al. Seasonality trends of Pediculosis capitis and *Phthirus pubis* in a young adult population: Follow-up of 20 years. *J Eur Acad Dermatol Venereol*. 2002;16:257–59.
17. Burkhart CG, Burkhart CN. Oral ivermectin for *Phthirus pubis*. *J Am Acad Dermatol*. 2004;51:1037; author reply 8.
18. Lacarrubba F, Micali G. The not-so-naked eye: Phthiriasis palpebrarum. *Am J Med*. 2013;126:960–61.
19. Schwartz RA, Altman R. Piedra. Medscape Reference. Updated May 05, 2015. Available at: http://emedicine.medscape.com/article/1092330-overview.
20. Schwartz RA: Superficial fungal infections. *Lancet*. 2004;364:1173–82.
21. Chuh A, Lee A, Wong W, et al. Diagnosis of Pediculosis pubis: A novel application of digital epiluminescence dermatoscopy. *J Eur Acad Dermatol Venereol*. 2007;21:837–38.
22. Zalaudek I, Argenziano G. Images in clinical medicine. Dermoscopy of nits and pseudonits. *N Engl J Med*. 2012;367:1741.
23. Yoon KC, Park HY, Seo MS, Park YG. Mechanical treatment of phthiriasis palpebrarum. *Korean J Ophthalmol*. 2003;17:71–73.

4 Parasitoses
Therapeutic monitoring of scabies and pediculosis

Giuseppe Micali, Aurora Tedeschi, Francesco Lacarrubba, and Dennis P. West

A great pitfall for scabies and pediculosis therapeutic studies to date is that primary and secondary study outcomes are indirectly assessed (presence or absence of live parasites, including eggs, determined by gross clinical inspection) and data are nonstandardized (highly variable) relative to time of therapeutic application. Certainly, kill times and kill rates are rarely determined or reported. Indeed, meta-analyses of randomized, controlled clinical trials for these parasitoses are scarce and, by nature, analyses are based on highly variable assessment methodology and data collection, followed by highly variable interpretation and reporting.[1–2]

Considering these significant limitations in efficacy studies to date for both scabies and pediculosis, Table 4.1 reports a combined subjective and objective relative assessment of efficacy and safety to provide a current guide to benefit-to-risk ratio for selected agents reported to be used in scabies and/or pediculosis.

Previous studies demonstrated that videodermatoscopy (VD) is a very effective and sensitive diagnostic tool for some cutaneous parasitoses, in particular scabies and pediculosis.[3–5] An important advantage of VD is its high compliance, as it does not cause pain or physical discomfort. For these reasons, VD seems to be a useful technique for evaluation of response to therapy, especially in those cases in which itch persists after treatment or patient compliance is doubtful. Based on these considerations, some studies have been conducted to evaluate VD's ability to monitor efficacy of scabies and pediculosis treatment and whether it allows determination of the optimal timing of drug application.

The use of VD in the therapeutic monitoring of scabies and pediculosis may provide enormous advantages in the quest to establish reproducible quantitative methodology for efficacy studies in these parasitoses.

THERAPEUTIC MONITORING OF SCABIES

Topical and systemic agents are quite effective in killing and eradicating the parasite (Table 4.1). Pruritus may increase and persist for up to 2 weeks after successful treatment due to continuing reactivity to substances released from the dying mites. Patients need to be reassured that itching is not always indicative of infestation after treatment. Pruritus lasting longer than 2 weeks after treatment may indicate treatment failure or resistance. Generally, a repeat treatment is given 7 days after the initial treatment to ensure that hatching larvae are destroyed.[6] Bed linens and towels should be washed after treatment, and areas of frequent body contact such as carpets, chairs, and sofas should be vacuumed.[7] It is important to treat close physical contact, even if asymptomatic, as well as the infested patient to minimize the risk of reinfestation.

The first study[8] to assess the use of epiluminescence light microscopy (ELM) for monitoring antiscabietic therapy was performed in 2001. The authors examined the mite's

TABLE 4.1
Combined subjective and objective relative assessment of reported efficacy and safety to provide a benefit-to-risk ratio category for selected agents used in scabies and/or pediculosis

Agent	Condition	Benefit: Risk
Benzyl alcohol Topical	pediculosis	1
Dimethicone Topical	pediculosis	1
Ivermectin Topical	pediculosis	1
Ivermectin Systemic	scabies and pediculosis	1
Malathion/terpineols combination therapy (US) Topical	scabies and pediculosis	1
Permethrin Topical	scabies and pediculosis	1
Benzyl benzoate Topical	scabies and pediculosis	2
Cotrimoxazole (trimethoprim/sulfamethoxazole) Systemic	pediculosis	2
Crotamiton Topical	scabies and pediculosis	2
Lindane Topical	scabies and pediculosis	2
Malathion monotherapy (UK) Topical	scabies and pediculosis	2
Petrolatum/mineral oil/vegetable (e.g., olive) oils Topical	pediculosis	2
Pyrethrins/piperonyl butoxide Topical	pediculosis	2
Sulfur Topical	scabies	2
Albendazole Systemic	pediculosis	3
Carbaryl Topical	pediculosis	3
Citronella Topical	pediculosis	3
Levamisole Systemic	pediculosis	3
Butter/margarine/mayonnaise Topical	pediculosis	na
Kerosene/gasoline/petroleum distillates Topical	pediculosis	na

1   *benefit/risk balanced*
2   *benefit/risk decreased*
3   *benefit/risk marginal*
na   *benefit/risk not acceptable*

morphological changes *in vivo*, the temporal progression of these changes, and their effectiveness as criteria for treatment. Twenty patients affected by scabies were observed: 7 patients received 12 mg of ivermectin as a single dose and 13 patients were treated with lindane or benzyl benzoate for 3 days. ELM was performed using ×8.25 and ×20.8 magnification. Before treatment, the average number of adult female mites on both hands and feet of all patients was 8.2. Epimeres (chitinous internal structures attached to legs), anterior outline, eating tools, and both pairs of forelegs and hind legs of *Sarcoptes scabiei* were observed. One week after treatment, the average number of adult female mites had dropped to 5.0. After 2 weeks, the animals began to degrade, and their outlines disappeared gradually; however, epimeres were even more distinct, especially in children. A granular hem was noticed in some cases. After 3 weeks, structures had progressively broken down or were missing. Statistically, no differences were found between patients treated orally and those treated locally. After 4 weeks, there were no visible remains. The authors suggested the decreasing number of mites might have resulted from both scratching and the renewal process of the corneal layer itself. Once the mite was dead, it was slowly promoted upward under a progressively thinning cover; this explained why the durable chitinous epimeres became even more distinct with time. The progressive degradation of its other, less durable components and its gradually disappearing outline suggested that the mite had degraded rather than simply been scratched away. Probably, the granular hem was a product of catabolism resulting from treatment.

Another study[9] evaluated a group of patients affected by scabies undergoing topical treatment with a thermo-labile foam of pyrethrins (0.165%) synergized with piperonyl butoxide (1.65%) to determine if VD would enhance monitoring of the clinical response to treatment and to determine if this technique would indicate the optimal timing of drug application. Twenty patients (12 male, 8 female; age 1–65 years) affected by scabies (diagnosis confirmed by VD) and who were treatment-naïve were included in the study. The foam was applied to the entire body, once at bedtime for two consecutive days. To detect treatment response, VD evaluation (Hi-Scope KH-2200 [Hirox Co. Ltd., Tokyo, Japan] equipped with a zoom lens that allows skin observation with incidental light at magnifications ranging from ×20 to ×600) of two selected skin areas for each patient was performed at baseline, 12, 24, 36, and 48 hours. At 48 hours, skin of the selected areas was scraped, followed by microscopic observation. In all patients, VD showed mite migration within burrows at 12 hours. At 24 hours, there was no evidence of active mite migration; at that time point most patients reported that itching symptoms had subsided. At 48 hours, the mites were generally no longer appreciable and an amorphous material, probably resulting from mite decomposition, was generally detectable at one end of an empty burrow (Figure 4.1). At this time, skin scraping followed by microscopic observation showed only mite remnants in all patients. None of the 20 patients showed evidence of infestation at a 2-week follow-up. VD confirmed that the foam was effective in the management of scabies, killing the mites at about 24 hours, when their immobilization could be established. In this study, the use of high magnification (up to ×600) allowed early recognition of the mite death.

In another single-arm multicenter study[10] including adults and children from 3 months of age with proven scabies, a 5% permethrin cream formulation was tested. In this study the evaluation of efficacy was performed with the stereo epiluminescence microscope of Kreusch (Fa. Wolfgang Kocher Feinmechanik, Mössingen, Germany, or a comparable device of another manufacturer) or with a videomicroscope with ×20–×60 magnification.

In conclusion, VD enhances the monitoring of clinical response to treatment and allows determination of the optimal timing of drug application. This may be particularly important in minimizing the risk of overtreatment, reducing the potential for side effects, and enhancing patient compliance.[11]

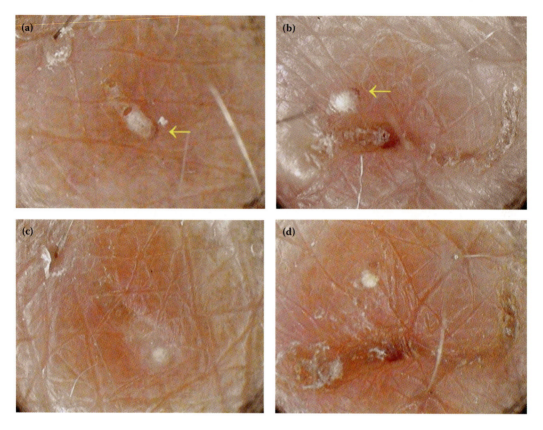

FIGURE 4.1 Treatment of scabies with pyrethrins + piperonyl butoxide. (a, b) VD evaluation showing the presence of Sarcoptes scabiei (arrows) at baseline. (c, d) After 48 hours of treatment the mites were no longer appreciable (×100).

THERAPEUTIC MONITORING OF PEDICULOSIS

A high percentage of cases of head lice are treated without medical supervision and with products that may be prone to overuse, leading to increased risk of developing resistance to such products. Resistance to virtually all topical products for treatment of pediculosis has been reported.[12–14] While treatment failure may be due to resistance in some cases, noncompliance or underuse of medication should always be considered. Whether changing treatment product or applying additional doses, the importance of consultation and patient education should be emphasized.[15] Some causes of treatment failure may be related to misdiagnosis or reinfestation. Usually an initial treatment is followed by a second application after 7–10 days to ensure that any hatching nymphs are destroyed.[16]

Pediculosis is usually treated with topical compounds with insecticidal activity (pyrethrin, permethrin, and malathion), with so-called natural products with mechanical action (e.g., essential oils), or with systemic drugs, such as antibiotics (trimetroprim) or ivermectin.[17] However, for many of these products, data about their real therapeutic efficacy or rapidity of action are not readily available. Moreover, evaluation methods have been based on very simplistic criteria (i.e., clinical examination before and after treatment).

VD can be used as a diagnostic tool in head and pubic lice infestation: it permits an easy identification of parasite and nits when these are not easy to identify with the naked eye.[18] The differentiation between vital and empty nits provides useful information about therapeutic response.

An *in vivo* study[18] was performed by means of a noncontact handheld dermatoscope (Dermlite; 3Gen, LLC). An 8-year old boy affected by *Pediculus capitis* was treated with permethrin 1% according to established protocols. One week after the first treatment cycle, dermatoscopic follow-up still revealed the presence of dark brown eggs containing nymphs, and two additional therapeutic cycles were performed. At the last visit, 3 weeks after diagnosis, no nits were observed and treatment was discontinued. In this case, the dermatoscopic examination allowed a safe and reliable differentiation of eggs containing nymphs from the empty cases of hatched louses and also from amorphous pseudo-nits. The characteristic dermatoscopic features not only let the authors establish a rapid diagnosis, but also were useful for the treatment monitoring, because vital eggs were still present after the first treatment cycle. Therefore, *in vivo* dermatoscopy may replace the more time-consuming *ex vivo* microscopic examination of the affected hairs in the daily routine.[18]

In our experience, VD allowed therapeutic monitoring with mercurial ointment in a case of phthiriasis palpebrarum. After 5 days of treatment, VD showed the persistence of few full nits not visible to the naked eye (Figure 4.2).

VD allows an *in vivo* evaluation of the movements and physiology of lice and eggs. Isolation of an adult parasite allows one to observe the louse and to prove its viability in *ex vivo* conditions (by means of a Petri dish). Through the isolation of *Pediculus humanus capitis* and through VD evaluation, it also is possible to assess the efficacy and rapidity of pediculocidal activity of topical pediculocides.

In 2006 a study was performed[19] with VD about the pediculocidal efficacy and rapidity of action of two different products indicated in the treatment of head lice. A formulation of synergized pyrethrin in thermophobic foam (Milice; Mipharm) was compared to a coconut and aniseed oil–based spray, with a mechanical action obtained by suffocation (Paranix; Chefaro). Ten experiments were performed on the same number of adults' specimens of *Pediculus humanus capitis* taken in three subjects with head lice infestation using a fine-tooth comb. Each louse was placed in a Petri dish with gauze on the bottom to improve the VD visualization (Hirox Hi-Scope KH-2200 equipped with lenses allowing magnifications ranging from ×20–×600). An initial observation of 180-second duration was performed to evaluate movements and peristaltic intestinal activity (that is visible in transparency) as an indicator of lice viability. After this time, a minimal quantity of pyrethrin thermophobic foam was applied on 5 parasites; the oil-based spray was applied on the other 5 parasites. The parasites' activity was then observed and recorded for 120 continuous minutes. In the case of the pyrethrin thermophobic foam product, in all performed tests, the absence of parasite movements was observed within 10 seconds of the contact with the product; the absence of peristalsis was noted within 60 seconds, and this finding was interpreted as mite death. With coconut and aniseed oil–based spray,

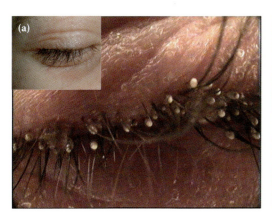
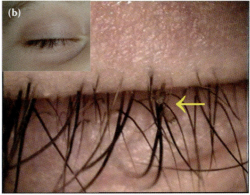

FIGURE 4.2 Treatment of phthiriasis palpebrarum with a mercurial ointment. (a) VD of lice and nits at baseline. (b) VD after 5 days of treatment: persistence of few full nits not visible to the naked eye (×30).

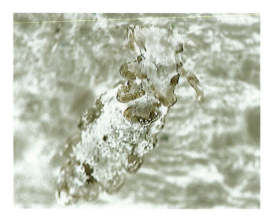

FIGURE 4.3 VD of an adult specimen of *Pediculus humanus* treated with the application of a topical compound that acts through a mechanical "choking" action (×80).

the lice also were alive after a continuous observation of 120 minutes after the application of the product. (On the spray's packaging, the time for optimal product activity is indicated as approximately 15 minutes.)

Successively, another similar preliminary study was performed from the group with a topical compound that acts through a mechanical action of "choking" the mite within few minutes (Figure 4.3).

In conclusion, VD represents a valid research tool for the evaluation of efficacy and time of action of topical pediculocides.[11] A further and future use of this tool could be represented by the study of possible lice resistance to commonly used substances with pediculocidal activity to contribute to the identification of alternative and appropriate therapeutic options.

REFERENCES

1. Hu S, Bigby M. Treating scabies: Results from an updated Cochrane review. *Arch Dermatol.* 2008;144:1638–40.
2. Burkhart CN, Burkhart CG. Recommendation to standardize pediculicidal and ovicidal testing for head lice (Anoplura: Pediculidae). *J Med Entomol.* 2001;38:127–29.
3. Argenziano G, Fabbrocini G, Delfino M. Epiluminescence microscopy. A new approach to *in vivo* detection of *Sarcoptes scabiei*. *Arch Dermatol.* 1997;133:751–53.
4. Micali G, Lacarrubba F, Lo Guzzo G. Scraping versus videodermatoscopy for the diagnosis of scabies: A comparative study. *Acta Derm Venereol.* 2000;79:396.
5. Lacarrubba F, Musumeci ML, Caltabiano R, et al. High-magnification videodermatoscopy: A new noninvasive diagnostic tool for scabies in children. *Pediatr Dermatol.* 2001;18:439–41.
6. Orkin M, Maibach HI. Scabies treatment: current considerations. *Curr Prob Dermatol.* 1996;24:151–56.
7. Elston DM. Controversies concerning the treatment of lice and scabies. *J Am Acad Dermatol.* 2002;46:794–96.
8. Haas N, Sterry W. The use of ELM to monitor the success of antiscabietic treatment. *Arch Dermatol.* 2001;137:1656–57.
9. Micali G, Lacarrubba F, Tedeschi A. Videodermatoscopy enhances the ability to monitor efficacy of scabies treatment and allows optimal timing of drug application. *J Eur Acad Dermatol.* 2004;18:153–54.
10. Hamm H, Beiteke U, Höger PH, et al. Treatment of scabies with 5% permethrin cream: Results of a German multicenter study. *J Dtsch Dermatol Ges.* 2006;4:407–13.
11. Micali G, Tedeschi A, West DP, et al. The use of videodermatoscopy to monitor treatment of scabies and pediculosis. *J Dermatolog Treat.* 2011;22:133–37.
12. Burkhart CG, Burkhart CN. Clinical evidence of lice resistance to over-the-counter products. *J Cutan Med Surg.* 2000;4:199–201.
13. Pollack RJ, Kiszewski A, Armstrong P, et al. Differential permethrin susceptibility of head lice sampled in the United States and Borneo. *Arch Pediatr Adolesc Med.* 1999;153:969–73.
14. Downs AM, Stafford KA, Harvey I, et al. Evidence for double resistance to permethrin and malathion in head lice. *Br J Dermatol.* 1999;141:508–11.
15. Chosidow O. Scabies and Pediculosis. *Lancet.* 2000;355:819–26.
16. Frankowski BL, Weiner LB. Head lice. *Pediatrics* 2002;110:638-43.
17. Dodd CS. Interventions for treating head-lice. *Cochrane Database Syst Rev.* 2001;2:CDOO1165.
18. Di Stefani A, Hofmann-Wellenhof R, Zalaudek I. Dermoscopy for diagnosis and treatment monitoring of pediculosis capitis. *J Am Acad Dermatol.* 2006;54:909–11.
19. Lacarrubba F, Nardone B, Milani M, et al. Head lice: *Ex vivo* videodermatoscopy evaluation of the pediculocidal activity of two different topical products. *G Ital Dermatol Venereol.* 2006;141:233–35.

5 Parasitoses
Tungiasis

Elvira Moscarella, Leonardo Spagnol Abraham, and Giuseppe Argenziano

DEFINITION

Tungiasis is an ectoparasitic disease caused by the burrowing flea *Tunga penetrans* or related species.[1]

EPIDEMIOLOGY/ETIOPATHOGENESIS

The flea has many common names, including the chigger flea, sand flea, chigoe, jigger, nigua, pigue, or bicho-de-pé, and is endemic in some parts of South and Central America, Africa, Asia, and the Caribbean. Data on tungiasis prevalence are variable and are not always available, especially for Africa. Tungiasis is reported to be very frequent in Trinidad with prevalence varying from 15.7% to 31.4%.[1–2] In a study conducted in a rural community in Lagos, the prevalence was 45.2%.[3] A surveillance performed in communities of lower socioeconomic status of northeast Brazil has demonstrated prevalence rates of up to 54.5% among the residents of such areas.[4] Only one autochthon case has been reported in Europe[5] and the disease is rarely diagnosed in North America, but it should no longer be obscure to physicians because of increasing international travel to tropical destinations. A study analyzed the most common locally endemic infections that travelers encounter visiting Brazil. The most common travel-related illnesses were dermatologic conditions (40%), diarrheal syndromes (25%), and febrile systemic illness (19%), and the most common dermatologic conditions were cutaneous larva migrans, myiasis, and tungiasis.[6] Travelers to affected countries must be advised to wear shoes (not sandals) when walking in rural areas in affected regions.

Tunga penetrans is a ground flea that infests the skin of humans and can have various animals (pigs, cows, cats, dogs, and rats) serving as usual reservoirs.[7–8] The disease is usually acquired by walking barefoot in humid ground contaminated by the flea. Therefore, the feet are the preferred site of penetration. The flea is not able to jump high; even so, ectopic lesions have been reported in almost all parts of the body and are associated with high infestation grades and young age.[9] Both male and female fleas may penetrate the skin, but after copulation, the male dies, whereas the female remains in the skin completing her vital cycle that lasts about 4–6 weeks. The flea penetrates the skin with the head of the exoskeleton, creating a cavity that reaches the superficial dermis, where it is nourished by the blood of the dermal vascular plexus. After penetration into the skin, the female starts producing eggs and enlarging her body from 1 mm to about 1 cm in diameter. Eggs and feces are eliminated through a small opening in the epidermis and then the flea dies in the cavity. The natural history of the disease has been divided into five phases:[10] (1) penetration, (2) hypertrophy, (3) the white halo phase, (4) inoculation, and (5) rest of the fleas in the host's cutis.

CLINICAL PRESENTATION/DIAGNOSIS

Tungiasis typically presents multiple, confluent, roundish papules or nodules located on the feet. The lesions are white-gray-yellowish in color and exhibit a small, central, brown opening. Penetration of the flea is asymptomatic or may be followed by an itching sensation. When the parasite enlarges its diameter, an inflammatory process causes pain to the host,[11] that is sometimes reported as very intense and debilitating.

The diagnosis is essentially clinical in endemic areas. In nonendemic areas, the lesion is usually single and can be easily misdiagnosed and confused with several other diseases like viral warts, foreign body reaction, fungal and bacterial infections, tumors, myiasis, and vasculitis. Early diagnosis and correct therapy are crucial to avoid frequent complications that may be caused by bacterial super-infections.[12]

Histopathologic examination reveals hyperkeratosis and acanthosis of the epidermis. The flea is located between the epidermis and the superficial dermis, embedded in a pseudocystic cavity that presents a small opening through which eggs and feces are expelled. An inflammatory perilesional infiltrate that is constituted by lymphocytes, neutrophils, and eosinophils is also present.

DERMATOSCOPY/ VIDEODERMATOSCOPY FEATURES

Physicians frequently see traveling-associated dermatoses with which they are not very familiar.[13] In this scenario, dermatoscopy can facilitate the early diagnosis of tropical dermatoses including tungiasis, thus leading to a correct approach (Figure 5.1).

Bauer and colleagues[14–15] first described the dermatoscopic aspects of tungiasis, identifying the dark spot as a pigmented ring with a central pore. This corresponds to the pigmented chitin surrounding the posterior opening of the flea exoskeleton. Di Stefani and colleagues[16] found a dermatoscopic gray-blue blotch, which they inferred to be related to developing eggs. The direct identification of eggs by dermatoscopy has been described by Cabrera's team.[17] After the flea reaches the dermis, by sequential and careful shaving of the epidermis and gently compresses the edges of the wound, a jelly-like bag emerges, which is visible as a bag full of eggs during dermatoscopy. Bakos et al.[18] described a further dermatoscopic feature defined as "whitish chains." They visualized the presence of whitish structures in a chain-like distribution perfectly matching *in vivo* with the jelly bag described by Cabrera's team[17,19] Dunn and colleagues[20] utilized *ex vivo* dermatoscopy for diagnosis confirmation. In their report, *in vivo* dermatoscopy revealed an annular brown ring with a central black pore. A diagnosis of tungiasis was suspected and management initiated immediately. This involved careful dissection of the stratum corneum before shelling out the intact flea, thus allowing the visualization, by *ex vivo* dermatoscopy, of the flea head on a distended "jelly sac" abdomen full of eggs.

Dermatoscopy can also allow a rapid differential diagnosis[21] with plantar warts and pigmented melanocytic lesions (a case of tungiasis simulating acral melanoma has been described).[7] In viral warts, the diagnosis is based on the presence of a verrucous, yellowish unstructured area exhibiting a variable number of irregularly distributed, red, brown, or black dots or linear streaks caused by chronic high vascular pressure at plantar sites. Pigmented acral melanoma can also be easily differentiated for the presence of specific dermatoscopic features such as the parallel ridge pattern.

In conclusion, clinical history, examination findings, and *in vivo* dermatoscopy are important clues for the diagnosis of tungiasis. After extraction of the intact parasite, the diagnosis can be confirmed by *ex vivo* dermatoscopy revealing the parasite's head and abdomen full of eggs (Figure 5.2).[20,22]

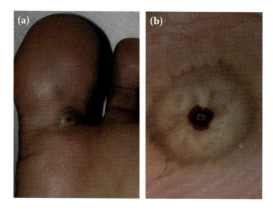

FIGURE 5.1 Tungiasis. (a) White-grey-yellowish round papule located on the foot. (b) At dermatoscopy, the lesion appears as white to light brown, with a central brownish opening corresponding to the posterior part of the flea's exoskeleton; gray-blue blotches can also be seen and represent the intestinal part of the flea (×10).

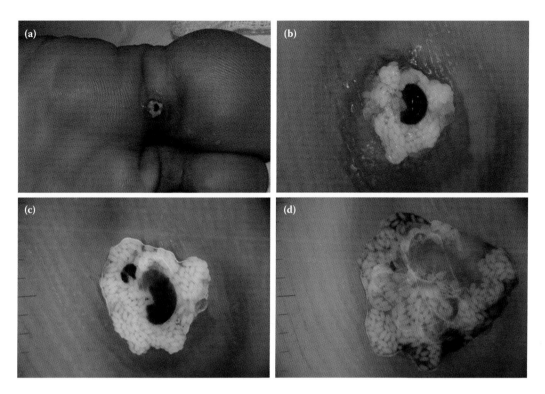

FIGURE 5.2 Sequential pictures of the procedure to remove the tungiasis flea. (a) Clinical aspect of the tunga after careful dissection of the stratum corneum before shelling out the intact flea. (b) *Ex vivo* dermatoscopy without contact showing numerous "rice-like" whitish structures corresponding to the eggs, and a black elongated structure in the middle, corresponding to the clotted blood. (c, d) Contact dermatoscopy with little pressure (c) and high pressure (d), showing the eggs within the clotted blood (×10).

REFERENCES

1. Chadee DD. Distribution patterns of tunga penetrans within a community in Trinidad, West Indies. *Trop Med Hyg.* 1994;97:167–70.
2. Chadee DD. Tungiasis among five communities in south western Trinidad, West Indies. *Ann Trop Med Parassitol.* 1998;92:107–13.
3. Ugnomoiko US, Ofoezie IE, Heukelbach J. Tungiasis: High prevalence, parasite load, and morbidity in a rural community in Lagos State, Nigeria. *Int J Dermatol.* 2007;46:475–81.
4. Heukelbach J, Costa AML, Wilckle T, et al. The animal reservoir of tunga penetrans in severely affected communities of north-east Brazil. *Med Vet Entomol.* 2004;18:329–35.
5. Veraldi S, Carrera C, Schianchi R. Tungiasis had reached Europe. *Dermatology.* 2000; 201:382.
6. Wilson ME, Chen LH, Han PV, et al.; GeoSentinel Surveillance Network. Illness in Travelers Returned From Brazil: The GeoSentinel Experience and Implications for the 2014 FIFA World Cup and the 2016 Summer Olympics. *Clin Infect Dis.* 2014;58(10):1347–56.
7. Franck S, Feldmeier H, Heukelbach J. Tungiasis: More than an exotic nuisance. *Travel Med Infect Dis.* 2003;1:159–66.
8. Kimpel S, Mehlhorn H, Heukelbach J, et al. Field trial of the efficacy of a combination of imidacloprid and permetrin against Tunga penetrans (sand flea, jigger flea) in dogs in Brazil. *Parassitol Res.* 2005;97:S113–19.
9. Heukelbach J, Wicke T, Eisele M, Feldmeier H. Ectopic localization of tungiasis. *Am J Trop Med Hyg.* 2002;67:214–16.
10. Eisele M, Heukelbach J, Van Marck E, et al. Investigations on the biology, epidemiology, pathology and control of Tunga penetrans in Brazil: I. Natural history of tungiasis in man. *Parasitol Res.* 2003;9(2):87–99.
11. Van Bruskirk C, Burd EM, Lee M. A painful, draining black lesion on the right heel. Tungiasis. *Clin Infect Dis.* 2006;43:65–66.

12. Feldmeier H, Heukelbach J, Eisele M, et al. Bacterial super-infection in human tungiasis. *Trop Med Int Health*. 2002;7:559–64.
13. Caumes E, Carriere J, Guermonprez G, et al. Dermatosis associated with travel to tropical countries: A prospective study of the diagnosis and management of 269 patients presenting to a tropical disease unit. *Clin Infect Dis*. 1995;20:542–48.
14. Bauer J, Forschner A, Garbe C, Rocken M. Dermoscopy of tungiasis. *Arch Dermatol*. 2004;140(6):761–63.
15. Bauer J, Forschner A, Garbe C, Rocken M. Variability of dermoscopic features of tungiasis. *Arch Dermatol*. 2005;141(5):643–44.
16. Di Stefani A, Rudolph CM, Hofmann-Wellnhof R, Mullegger RR. An additional dermoscopic feature of tungiasis. *Arch Dermatol*. 2005;141(8):1045–46.
17. Cabrera R, Daza F. Tungiasis: Eggs seen with dermoscopy. *Br J Dermatol*. 2008;158(3):635–66.
18. Bakos RM, Bakos L. "Whitish chains": A remarkable *in vivo* dermoscopic finding of tungiasis. *Br J Dermatol*. 2008,159: 991–92.
19. Cabrera R, Daza F. Dermoscopy in the diagnosis of tungiasis. *Br J Dermatol*. 2009;160(5):1136–37.
20. Dunn R, Asher R, Bowling J. Dermoscopy: *Ex vivo* visualization of fleas head and bag of eggs confirms the diagnosis of Tungiasis. *Australas J Dermatol*. 2012;53(2):120–22.
21. Zalaudek I, Giacomel J, Cabo H, et al. Entodermoscopy: A new tool for diagnosing skin infections and infestations. *Dermatology*. 2008;216(1):14–23.
22. Criado PR, Landman G, Reis VM, Belda W Jr. Tungiasis under dermoscopy: *In vivo* and *ex vivo* examination of the cutaneous infestation due to Tunga penetrans. *An Bras Dermatol*. 2013;88(4):649–51.

6 Parasitoses
Cutaneous larva migrans

Elvira Moscarella, Renato Bakos, and Giuseppe Argenziano

DEFINITION

Cutaneous larva migrans (CLM) is a cutaneous parasitosis characterized by one or more serpiginous lesions.[1–3] It is also known as "creeping eruption."

EPIDEMIOLOGY/ETIOPATHOGENESIS

CLM is endemic in tropical and subtropical geographic areas and the southwestern United States; however, the increased foreign travels by the world's population have no longer confined the parasitosis to these areas.[3–4]

CLM is caused by accidental percutaneous penetration and subsequent migration of larvae of various animal hookworms (helmints). *Ancylostoma braziliense* is the most common parasite implicated in the development of CLM.[2] Its length and width are approximately 650 and 20 μm, respectively. Eggs are shed in feces of infested dogs and cats, hatch in the superficial layer of the soil, and then develop into larvae.[1–2] Upon close contact, the larvae penetrate human skin. The larvae cannot penetrate the basement membrane of human skin and remain confined to the epidermis. This results in the development of serpiginous skin lesions.

CLINICAL PRESENTATION/DIAGNOSIS

The disease manifests as an erythematous, serpiginous, pruritic, cutaneous eruption. Lesions are typically distributed on the distal lower extremities, including the dorsa of the feet and the interdigital spaces of the toes, but can also occur in the anogenital region, the buttocks, the hands, and the knees. The diagnosis of CLM is primarily based on the classic clinical appearance of the eruption. Only a minority of patients demonstrate systemic involvement, such as peripheral eosinophilia and increased immunoglobulin E (IgE) levels on total serum immunoglobulin determinations. A skin biopsy sample in CLM, taken just ahead of the leading edge of a tract, may show a larva (periodic acid-Schiff positive) in a suprabasal burrow, basal layer tracts, spongiosis with intraepidermal vesicles, necrotic keratinocytes, and an epidermal and upper dermal chronic inflammatory infiltrate with many eosinophils.[1–2]

Even though CLM is self-limited, the intense pruritus and risk for infection mandate treatment. Prevention involves avoidance of direct skin contact with fecally contaminated soil.

DERMATOSCOPY/ VIDEODERMATOSCOPY FEATURES

Dermatoscopy can be a helpful aid in the diagnosis of CLM (Figure 6.1), although its efficacy has not been adequately established. In a report by Elsner and colleagues,[5] the larva of CLM was detected by dermatoscopy at ×40 magnification, but in another study of 18 patients, the diagnosis of CLM was established by history and clinical examination, and only one larva was visualized within one lesion in one patient by dermatoscopy.[6] However, in this latter study dermatoscopy was limited to a standard ×10 magnification, which could account for the low sensitivity in detecting larva. Zalaudek and colleagues[7] described an additional case in which the characteristic clinical features and symptoms of CLM suggested the diagnosis. Nonetheless, dermatoscopy revealed translucent brownish structureless areas in a segmental arrangement, which corresponded to the body of the larva, while the empty burrow revealed dotted vessels.[7] In a report by Aljasser and colleagues, polarized dermatoscopy of the serpiginous tract showed two oval structures, each with a yellow periphery and brown center that may represent the body of the larva.[8]

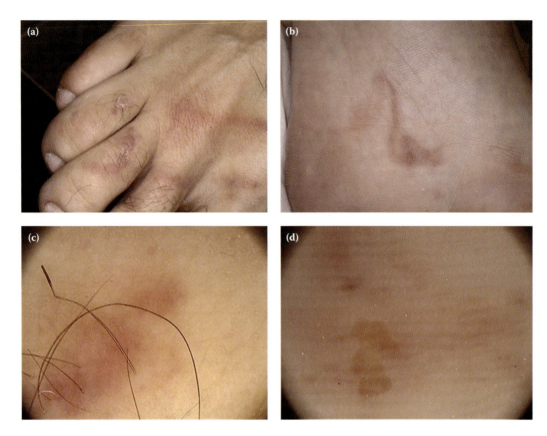

FIGURE 6.1 Two cases of cutaneous larva migrans occurring in two young Brazilian patients. (a, b) Erythematous raised serpiginous tract over the toes (a) and medial aspect of the right foot (b). (c, d) Dermatoscopy of the same cases revealing respectively a brownish homogeneous pigmentation (c) and a brownish to yellow structureless area that may correspond to the body of the larva (d) (×20).

In conclusion, the efficacy of dermatoscopy for the diagnosis of CLM has not been adequately established, and further reports, using both standard and high magnification, are needed.

REFERENCES

1. Feldmeier H, Schuster A. Mini review: Hookworm-related cutaneous larva migrans. *Eur J Clin Microbiol Infect Dis.* 2012; 31:915–18.
2. Le Joncour A, Lacour SA, Lecso G, et al. Molecular characterization of *Ancylostoma braziliense* larvae in a patient with hookworm-related cutaneous larva migrans. *Am J Trop Med Hyg.* 2012;86:843–45.
3. Wilson ME, Chen LH, Han PV, et al; GeoSentinel Surveillance Network. Illness in Travelers Returned From Brazil: The GeoSentinel Experience and Implications for the 2014 FIFA World Cup and the 2016 Summer Olympics. *Clin Infect Dis.* 2014;58(10):1347–56.
4. Edelglass JW, Douglass MC, Stiefler R, Tessler M. Cutaneous larva migrans in northern climates. A souvenir of your dream vacation. *J Am Acad Dermatol.* 1982;7(3):353–58.
5. Elsner E, Thewes M, Worret WI. Cutaneous larva migrans detected by epiluminescence microscopy. *Acta Derm Venereol.* 1997;77:487–88.
6. Veraldi S, Schianchi R, Carrera C. Epiluminescence microscopy in cutaneous larva migrans. *Acta Derm Venereol.* 2000;80:233.
7. Zalaudek I, Giacomel J, Cabo H, et al. Entodermoscopy: a new tool for diagnosing skin infections and infestations. *Dermatology.* 2008;216:14–23.
8. Aljasser MI, Lui H, Zeng H, Zhou Y. Dermoscopy and near-infrared fluorescence imaging of cutaneous larva migrans. *Photodermatol Photoimmunol Photomed.* 2013;29(6):337–38.

7 Parasitoses
Cutaneous leishmaniasis

Pedro Zaballos Diego

DEFINITION

Cutaneous leishmaniasis (CL) is a common protozoan infection caused by several species of the genus *Leishmania*.

EPIDEMIOLOGY/ETIOPATHOGENESIS

CL is widely distributed and is prevalent in Africa, the Middle East, Latin America, and Mediterranean areas.[1] *Leishmania* species causing the disease include *L donovani*, *L tropica*, *L aethiopica*, *L major*, and *L infantum*. They are obligatory intracellular protozoa and are transmitted by infected animals to humans through the bite of Phlebotomine sandflies in the old world or Lutzomya in the new world.[1] The epidemiological and clinical features of the disease vary significantly depending on the type of parasite, vectors, immune system of patients, and environmental conditions.

CLINICAL PRESENTATION/DIAGNOSIS

Clinically, CL usually presents as a small papule that can progress into an erythematous nodule or indurated scaly plaque or into ulcers with regular contours and a central crust, which often tends to be hemorrhagic. These lesions appear mainly on uncovered areas such as the face and limbs, after a period of incubation of a few weeks or months. The polymorphous clinical spectrum of CL commonly makes its clinical diagnosis difficult. Differential diagnosis involves a wide range of skin diseases, including bites, sarcoidosis, infectious diseases (foruncle, tuberculosis, leprosy, actinomycetoma, sporotrichosis), melanocytic lesions (Spitz/Reed nevi, amelanotic melanoma), skin cancer (basal cell carcinoma, squamous cell carcinoma, keratoacanthoma), pyogenic granuloma, and cutaneous metastasis.[1–6] The suspected clinical diagnosis is confirmed by the demonstration of amastigotes in infected skin, by the growth of promastigotes in cultures medium, or by polymerase chain reaction–based methods, which may not always be available in routine daily practice and are costly and time-consuming.[1–6]

DERMATOSCOPY/VIDEODERMATOSCOPY FEATURES

Dermatoscopy has demonstrated to be a useful technique to improve the diagnosis of CL (Figures 7.1–7.7), depending on the experience of the user and the type of skin lesion.[1–6]

The main dermatoscopic structures associated with CL were described by Llambrich and colleagues in 2009.[2] Later, teams led by Taheri (144 cases)[3] and Yücel (145 cases)[4] validated these findings in their countries and added some additional structures.

The most common findings are the presence of generalized erythema (82%–100% of cases) and vascular structures (87%–100%) that correspond to the presence of dilated and telangiectatic vessels in these lesions.[2–6] The range of vessels associated with CL is wide. Comma-shaped vessels were most commonly found in the study by Llambrich's team,[2] dotted vessels in the study by Taheri's team,[3] and linear irregular vessels in the study by Yücel's team.[4] In any case, comma-shaped vessels (4%–73%), linear irregular vessels (30%–57%), dotted vessels (16%–61%), polymorphous atypical vessels (3%–26%), hairpin vessels (17%–37.5%), arborizing telangiectasias (11%–36.5%), glomerular-like vessels (7%–23%), and corkscrew vessels (0%–7%) can be found.[2–4] However, as these vessels are seen in many other diseases, they do not have a definitive diagnostic value.

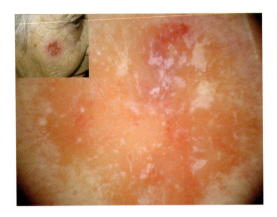

FIGURE 7.1 Dermatoscopy of cutaneous leishmaniasis: generalized erythema, vascular structures, scales, and some yellow tear-like structures (×10).

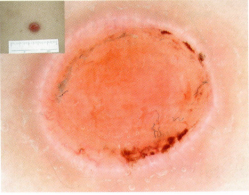

FIGURE 7.4 Dermatoscopy of cutaneous leishmaniasis: generalized erythema, vascular structures, hemorrhagic crusts, and an incipient white starbust-like pattern (×10).

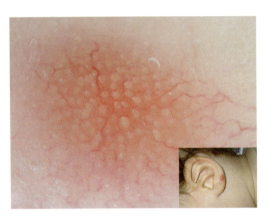

FIGURE 7.2 Dermatoscopy of cutaneous leishmaniasis: generalized erythema, vascular structures (mainly arborizing telangiectasias), and yellow tear-like structures (×10).

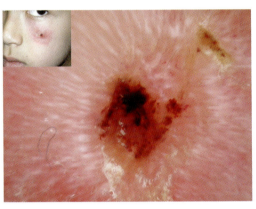

FIGURE 7.5 Dermatoscopy of cutaneous leishmaniasis in a child: generalized erythema, vascular structures, hemorrhagic crusts, and a remarkable white starbust-like pattern (×10).

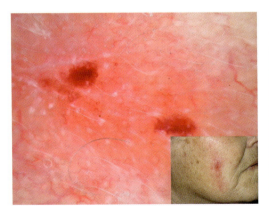

FIGURE 7.3 Dermatoscopy of cutaneous leishmaniasis in initial phase: generalized erythema and vascular structures (polymorphous atypical vessels) (×10).

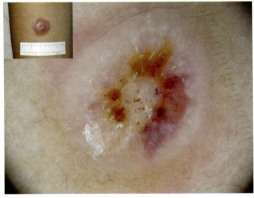

FIGURE 7.6 Dermatoscopy of cutaneous leishmaniasis in advanced phase: central erosion/ulceration combined with scales, white starbust-like pattern, and vascular structures at the periphery (×10).

Parasitoses

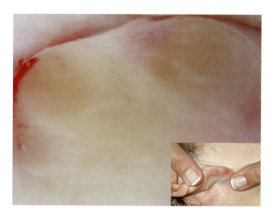

FIGURE 7.7 Dermatoscopy of cutaneous leishmaniasis located on the right ear of a 70-year-old woman: two large salmon-colored ovoid structures that are reminiscent of the apple jelly–like appearance seen in other granulomatous diseases on diascopy (×10).

The most remarkable and specific dermatoscopic features associated with CL are the yellow tear-like structures and the white starbust-like pattern. The yellow tear-like structures are roundish or oval ("tear drop form") white-yellowish structures that correspond to the follicular or keratin plugs. Llambrich and colleagues[2] found these yellow tears in 53% of cases, Yücei and colleagues[4] in 40% of cases, and Taheri and colleagues[3] in 41.7% of cases. These relatively high values may indicate that these structures are important dermatoscopic features of CL. The white starbust-like pattern corresponds histologically to the presence of parakeratotic hyperkeratosis and is located peripherally around central erosions or crusts. Llambrich's team[2] found this white starbust-like pattern in 38% of cases, Yücei's[4] in 18.6% of cases, and Taheri's[3] in 60.4% of cases. As this pattern has not been previously associated with other dermatological lesions, it may represent a valuable dermatoscopic criterion.

Other dermatoscopic structures that can be found in CL include salmon-colored ovoid structures, observed in 13% of cases in Yücei's series,[4] central erosions or ulcers (35%–46% of cases),[2–6] hyperkeratosis or scales (33%–50%),[2–6] yellow hue (43.8% of cases in Taheri's series),[3] milia-like cysts (4.9% of cases in Taheri's series),[3] and perilesional hypopigmented halo (2.8% of cases in Yücei's series).[4]

Llambrich and colleagues[2] identified two main dermatoscopic patterns of CL that correlate with the evolution of the lesions: in early cases, papular lesions are characterized by vascular structures and yellow tear-like structures; in more advanced cases, nodular lesions are characterized by central erosion/ulceration combined with scales, white starbust-like pattern, and vascular structures at the periphery.

REFERENCES

1. Reithinger R, Dujardin JC, Louzir H, et al. Cutaneous leishmaniasis. *Lancet Infect Dis.* 2007;7:581–96.
2. Llambrich A, Zaballos P, Terrasa F, et al. Dermoscopy of cutaneous leishmaniasis. *Br J Dermatol.* 2009;160:756–61.
3. Taheri AR, Pishgooei N, Maleki M, et al. Dermoscopic features of cutaneous leishmaniasis. *Int J Dermatol.* 2013;52:1361–66.
4. Yücel A, Günaşti S, Denli Y, Uzun S. Cutaneous leishmaniasis: New dermoscopic findings. *Int J Dermatol.* 2013;52:831–37.
5. Raone B, Raboni R, Ismaili A. Erythematous nodule of the left eyebrow in a 14-year-old boy. *JAMA Dermatol.* 2014;150:201–2.
6. Micali G, Lacarrubba F, Massimino D, Schwartz RA. Dermatoscopy: Alternative uses in daily clinical practice. *J Am Acad Dermatol.* 2011;64:1135–46.

8 Parasitoses
Trombiculiasis

Maria Rita Nasca and Giuseppe Micali

DEFINITION

Trombiculiasis is an infestation of the skin, also known as "chiggers," caused by the larval stage of different species belonging to the phylum Arthropoda, class Arachnida, subclass Acarina.[1–2]

EPIDEMIOLOGY/ETIOPATHOGENESIS

Neotrombicula autumnalis is the most prevalent species in the temperate and humid European environment, whereas *Trombicula alfreddugesi* is considered the most diffuse species in the Southeast and Midwest areas of North America. Adult individuals live and reproduce on the soil especially during warmer and wet late summer months. Eggs usually hatch at the end of autumn, about 10 days after deposition. New mites at their larval stage are obliged parasites of warm-blooded hosts, and usually feed and grow on small rodents and dogs' skin injecting lytic enzymes to digest cutaneous cells for 2–10 days before returning to the soil, where, after about 6 weeks, they first turn into nymphae and then into eight-legged adult individuals.[3–4]

CLINICAL PRESENTATION/DIAGNOSIS

Humans engaged in outdoor activities or staying in rural areas for professional or recreational purposes may become occasional hosts of this ectoparasitic infestation that is more common in autumn and should be suspected when dealing with subjects at risk (farmers, hunters, children, etc.) showing an itchy eruption. After climbing on the host, larvae usually move rapidly toward moist areas where skin is thinner and feeding is easier, such as the antecubital, axillary, popliteal, and inguinal grooves. They do not dig burrows but attach to the skin, more often settling on covered areas where clothes fit tightly, including the waist. Attachment itself is usually uneventful, but the injection of lytic enzymes through the feeding apparatus (stylosome) that follows a few hours later causes intense itch and onset of tiny spots of erythema on the affected areas. Scratching may easily cause detachment of the mite, which will not be able to attach again to the skin afterward. However, persistence of parts of the stylosome in the skin causes long-lasting pruritus, due to an immune inflammatory response, that subsides only several days later when the mite remnants are discarded through the skin. Pruritic wheals or papules usually ensue in previously sensitized individuals (Figure 8.1). Scratching marks and superinfection also frequently occur.[3–4]

Trombiculiasis is not considered rare but it is underreported and, probably, often misdiagnosed. Cutaneous findings are nonspecific, and an accurate anamnesis is essential to address this challenging diagnosis. Parasites may easily be missed or barely appreciable with common magnification lenses, so that their identification may be quite difficult.

DERMATOSCOPY/VIDEODERMATOSCOPY FEATURES

Videodermatoscopy is a useful tool for the diagnosis of ectoparasitic disorders.[5–6] In trombiculiasis it can easily reveal at ×30 magnification the characteristic reddish mite strongly attached to the patient's skin that may otherwise go overlooked (Figure 8.2a). Moreover, at ×150 magnification, details useful to recognize trombiculid mites in their larval stage and make a correct definitive diagnosis are easily appreciable (Figure 8.2b). They appear as 0.2–0.4 mm roundish and elongated orange mites with three

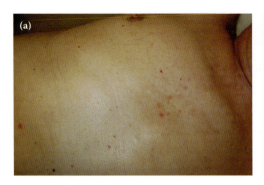
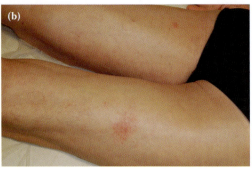

FIGURE 8.1 Trombiculiasis: wheals and papules on trunk (a) and legs (b).

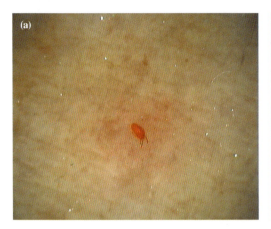
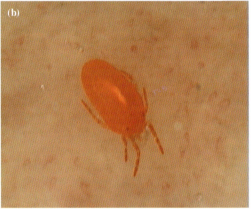

FIGURE 8.2 Dermatoscopy of the larval stage of trombiculid mite on the patient's skin at low (×30) (a) and high magnification (×150) (b).

pairs of long legs, two paired eyes, and a feeding apparatus with visible hooked chelicerae and segmented palps.[4] Such traits, common to larvae of several trombiculid mites, may be inadequate for a stringent taxonomic assignment but yet enable unequivocal identification of chigger mites in the medical setting.

No specific medications are required in the management of human trombiculiasis. Using repellants and avoiding exposure by wearing adequate clothing when accessing infested areas, along with accurate washing of body and clothes with soap and hot water immediately after, are usually effective prevention measures.[3–4]

REFERENCES

1. Stekolnikov AA, Santibáñez P, Palomar AM, Oteo JA. Neotrombicula inopinata (Acari: Trombiculidae)—A possible causative agent of trombiculiasis in Europe. *Parasit Vectors*. 2014;7:90.
2. Martens H, de Mendonça Melo M, van den Bosch W, van Genderen PJ. A "chigsaw" puzzle after a vacation in Brazil. *Neth J Med*. 2012;70(7):321–25.
3. Guarneri F, Pugliese A, Giudice E, et al. Trombiculiasis: clinical contribution. *Eur J Dermatol*. 2005;15(6):495–96.
4. Nasca MR, Lacarrubba F, Micali G. Diagnosis of trombiculosis by videodermatoscopy. *Emerg Infect Dis*. 2014;20(6):1059–60.
5. Micali G, Lacarrubba F, Massimino D, Schwartz RA. Dermatoscopy: Alternative uses in daily clinical practice. *J Am Acad Dermatol*. 2011;64(6):1135–46.
6. Zalaudek I, Giacomel J, Cabo H, et al. Entodermoscopy: A new tool for diagnosing skin infections and infestations. *Dermatology*. 2008;216(1):14–23.

9 Infectious diseases
Cutaneous and genital warts

Francesco Lacarrubba, Anna Elisa Verzì, Marco Ardigò, and Giuseppe Micali

Human papillomaviruses (HPVs) are DNA double-strand viruses that exhibit tropism for cells of the stratified squamous epithelium and that are associated with several cutaneous or mucosal benign and malignant lesions. To date, more than 100 different types of HPV have been identified.[1] Transmission may be direct or indirect. The most common clinical manifestations of HPV infection are represented by cutaneous and genital warts.

CUTANEOUS WARTS

DEFINITION

Cutaneous warts are benign epithelial keratinocytes proliferations that may affect any skin site, particularly the extremities.

EPIDEMIOLOGY/ETIOPATHOGENESIS

They are very common with an estimated incidence of 7%–10% in the European population and 1% in the US population.[2] Incidence increases 50–100 times in immunocompromised subjects, such as kidney-transplant patients.[3] HPV 1, 2, 3, 4, 7, 10, 27, and 57 are generally involved.

CLINICAL PRESENTATION/DIAGNOSIS

The clinical appearance of cutaneous warts is variable. *Common warts* (verrucae vulgaris) present as single or multiple, usually asymptomatic papules with a rough surface of varying sizes (Figure 9.1a). They may occur in any part of the integument but are more common on the back of hands and fingers. Morphological variants are represented by filiform warts, which are pedunculated, spiculated lesions that mainly affect the face and neck. *Palmo-plantar warts* may present as superficial, hyperkeratotic plaques, also called mosaic warts, or as deep, painful lesions, also known as myrmecia (Figure 9.2a). *Flat warts* (verrucae planae) are rounded or polygonal slightly raised papules, of skin color or pigmented (brownish, slightly yellowish), with a flat, smooth, or slightly rough surface (Figure 9.3a). They are commonly located on the face and the back of the hands, and they may be numerous with a linear distribution.

The diagnosis of cutaneous warts is usually based on typical clinical appearance.

DERMATOSCOPY/VIDEODERMATOSCOPY FEATURES

Dermatoscopy may be useful for a more accurate diagnosis. *Common warts* display multiple densely packed papillae, containing central red dotted vessels, which are surrounded by whitish halos (Figure 9.1b). Irregularly distributed, hemorrhagic reddish to black dots or streaks may be present.[4–7] *Palmo-plantar warts* reveal verrucous, yellowish structureless areas exhibiting multiple irregularly distributed red to brown to black dots or linear streaks due to hemorrhages (Figure 9.2b). These dots are helpful criteria to distinguish plantar warts from calluses, which lack blood spots.[8] Skin lines are typically interrupted.[9] *Flat warts* are characterized by regularly distributed, tiny red dots on a light-brown to yellow background (Figure 9.3b).[6–7] These features are helpful to distinguish them from acne comedones, which by contrast typically reveal a central white to yellow pore corresponding to the hair follicle opening.

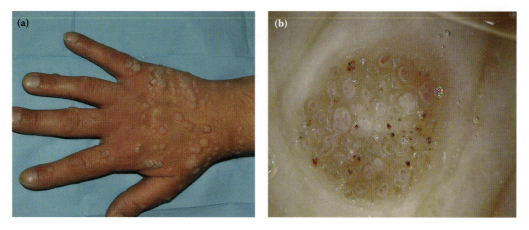

FIGURE 9.1 Common warts. (a) Clinical aspect. (b) Dermatoscopy showing multiple densely packed papillae, containing central red dotted vessels, which are surrounded by whitish halos (×30).

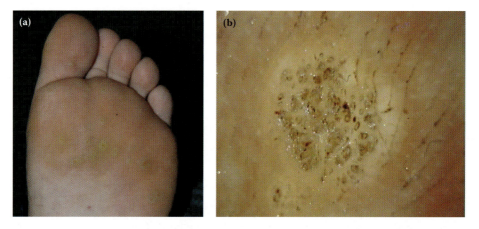

FIGURE 9.2 Plantar warts. (a) Clinical aspect. (b) Dermatoscopy showing a verrucous, yellowish structureless area exhibiting multiple irregularly distributed red to brown dots. Skin lines are interrupted (×30).

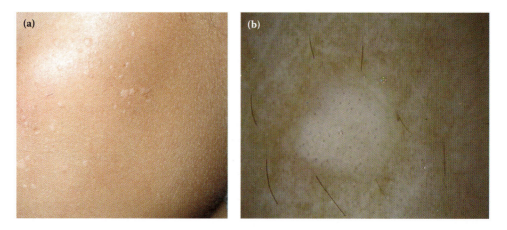

FIGURE 9.3 Flat warts. (a) Clinical aspect. (b) Dermatoscopy showing regularly distributed, tiny, red dots on a yellowish background (×30).

GENITAL WARTS

Definition

Genital warts or condylomata acuminata represent the genital and perigenital manifestation of HPV infection.

Epidemiology/Etiopathogenesis

Genital warts are widely diffused and represent the most frequent sexually transmitted infection in the Western world. They are frequently encountered from age 20–45, and men and women are equally affected.[10] HPV 6 and 11 are generally involved and are characterized by low risk of potential malignancy.

Clinical presentation/Diagnosis

Clinically, genital warts generally present as asymptomatic, pinkish, small papules (Figure 9.4a) or filiform, pedunculated, cauliflower-like lesions (Figure 9.5a). An accurate early diagnosis of genital warts is essential for prompt and correct management to avoid the spread of the disease. Clinical appearance, along with a history of acquired slowly enlarging papules, often allows an accurate diagnosis, unless there are single or unusual lesions that may mislead an otherwise straightforward clinical diagnosis. Application of 3%–5% acetic acid enhances diagnostic ability to some extent; however, this technique is considered nonspecific.[11] Histopathology, immunohistochemistry and polymerase chain reaction (PCR) techniques are generally confined to research as they are costly and time-consuming.

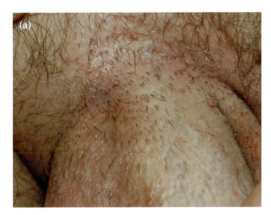
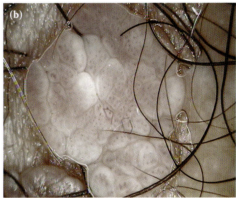

FIGURE 9.4 Papular genital warts. (a) Clinical aspect. (b) Dermatoscopy showing whitish network circumscribing areas centered by dilated glomerular vessels (×30).

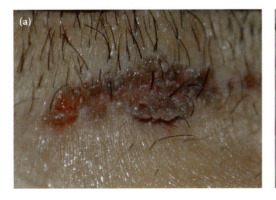
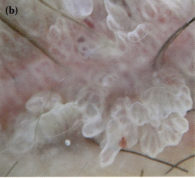

FIGURE 9.5 Cauliflower-like genital wart. (a) Clinical aspect. (b) Dermatoscopy showing multiple, irregular whitish projections arising from a common base and comprising elongated and dilated vessels (×30).

DERMATOSCOPY/VIDEODERMATOSCOPY FEATURES

Dermatoscopy is a useful technique for the diagnosis of genital warts. In papular lesions, it shows the presence of a whitish network circumscribing areas centered by dilated glomerular vessels (Figure 9.4b). In the case of the cauliflower-like genital warts, dermatoscopy shows in some areas of the lesions the same pattern of papular lesions; in other areas, generally at the periphery, multiple, irregular whitish projections arising from a common base and comprising elongated and dilated vessels may be observed (Figure 9.5b). Histopathologically, the whitish reticular network seen in papular lesions correlates with hyperkeratosis and acanthosis, and the glomerular vessels correspond to tortuous and dilated capillaries in the papillary dermis. The whitish projections typical of cauliflower-like lesions correspond to marked papillomatosis, hyperkeratosis, and acanthosis, and the dilated vessels seen at dermatoscopy correlate with those seen at microscopic observation along the elongated papillae.[7,12–15]

Dermatoscopy may help to differentiate anogenital warts from other genital growths such as pearly penile papules, Fordyce's spots, molluscum contagiosum, angiokeratoma of Fordyce, lymphangiomas, vestibular papillae, and lichen nitidus.[16]

For the evaluation of genital warts, the use of videodermatoscopy (VD) is much more preferable to the use of the handheld dermatoscope for higher magnification and resolution of distinguishing features. Moreover, VD technology eliminates the sometimes embarrassing situation of the physician having to place his or her head in close contact with the skin surface.

REFERENCES

1. Leto MD, Santos Júnior GF, Porro AM, Tomimori J. Human papillomavirus infection: Etiopathogenesis, molecular biology and clinical manifestations. *An Bras Dermatol.* 2011;86:306–17.
2. Hengge UR. Papillomavirus diseases. *Hautarzt.* 2004;55:841–51.
3. Lindelof B, Sigurgeirsson B, Gabel H, Stern RS. Incidence of skin cancer in 5356 patients following organ transplantation. *Br J Dermatol.* 2000;143:614–18.
4. Tanioka M, Nakagawa Y, Maruta N, Nakanishi G. Pigmented wart due to human papilloma virus type 60 showing parallel ridge pattern in dermoscopy. *Eur J Dermatol.* 2009;19:643–44.
5. Yoong C, Di Stefani A, Hofmann-Wellenhof R, et al. Unusual clinical and dermoscopic presentation of a wart. *Australas J Dermatol.* 2009; 50:228–29.
6. Vázquez-López F, Kreusch J, Marghoob AA. Dermoscopic semiology: Further insights into vascular features by screening a large spectrum of nontumoral skin lesions. *Br J Dermatol.* 2004;150:226–31.
7. Zalaudek I, Giacomel J, Cabo H, et al. Entodermoscopy: A new tool for diagnosing skin infections and infestations. *Dermatology.* 2008;216:14–23.
8. Kim HO, Bae JM, Kim YY, et al. Differential diagnosis of wart from callus and healed wart with aid of dermoscopy. *Dermatology.* 2006;212:307.
9. Lee D-Y, Park J-H, Lee J-H, et al. The use of dermoscopy for the diagnosis of plantar wart. *J Eur Acad Dermatol Venereol.* 2009;23:726–27.
10. Majewski S, Jablonska S. Human papillomaviruses-associated tumors of the skin and mucosa. *J Am Acad Dermatol.* 1997;36:658–59.
11. Kumar B, Gupta S. The acetowhite test in genital human papillomavirus infection in men: What does it add? *J Eur Acad Dermatol Venereol.* 2001;15:27–29.
12. Lacarrubba F, Dinotta F, Nasca MR, Micali G. Enhanced diagnosis of genital warts with videodermatoscopy: histopathologic correlation. *G Ital Dermatol Venereol.* 2012;147:215–16.
13. Dong H, Shu D, Campbell TM, et al. Dermatoscopy of genital warts. *J Am Acad Dermatol.* 2011;64:859–64.
14. Kim SH, Seo SH, Ko HC, et al. The use of dermatoscopy to differentiate vestibular papillae, a normal variant of the female external genitalia, from condyloma acuminata. *J Am Acad Dermatol.* 2009;60:353–55.
15. Watanabe T, Yoshida Y, Yamamoto O. Differential diagnosis of pearly penile papules and penile condyloma acuminatum by dermoscopy. *Eur J Dermatol.* 2010;20:414–15.
16. Micali G, Lacarrubba F. Augmented diagnostic capability using videodermatoscopy on selected infectious and non-infectious penile growths. *Int J Dermatol.* 2011;50:1501–5.

10 Infectious diseases
Molluscum contagiosum

Pedro Zaballos Diego

DEFINITION

Molluscum contagiosum (MC) is an infectious disease caused by a poxvirus of the *Molluscipox virus* genus. It was first described by Bateman in the beginning of the 19th century.

EPIDEMIOLOGY/ETIOPATHOGENESIS

There are four main subtypes of MC virus (MCV): MCV I, MCV II, MCV III, and MCV IV. There is no apparent relationship between viral subtype, morphology, or anatomical distribution. However, there appears to be marked geographical variation in the distribution of subtypes. The disease is transmitted primarily through direct skin contact with an infected individual. Fomites have been suggested as another source of infection. MCV can be found worldwide with a higher distribution in tropical areas and has a higher incidence in children, sexually active adults, and immunocompromised subjects. The average incubation time is between 2 and 7 weeks with a range extending to 6 months.

CLINICAL PRESENTATION/DIAGNOSIS

Clinically, MC presents as an eruption of multiple papules. The morphology of an individual lesion is a dome-shaped, flesh colored, or pearly papule with an umbilicated center (Figures 10.1–10.2). Lesions vary in size from 1–10 mm, although occasionally giant lesions are seen. The papules may be atypical in size, shape, and color, and signs of inflammation may occur spontaneously or after trauma. The lesions are often grouped in small areas but also may become widely disseminated. Any cutaneous surface may be involved, but favored sites include the axillae, the antecubital and popliteal fossae, and the crural folds in children. Autoinoculation is common. MC in adults affects the groin, genital area, thighs, and lower abdomen and is often acquired with sexual intercourse. Histologically, MC exhibits epidermal hyperplasia producing a crater filled with huge (up to 35 microns) eosinophilic to basophilic intracytoplasmatic inclusions that are called molluscum bodies or Henderson-Patterson bodies. MC is a self-limited disease, which if left untreated will eventually resolve in immunocompetent hosts but may persist in atopic and immunocompromised individuals.[1–5]

The clinical diagnosis of MC is usually easy, mainly in pediatric patients, because the lesions are normally characteristic in appearance. However, MC may be occasionally confused with other lesions, particularly in adulthood.[6]

DERMATOSCOPY/ VIDEODERMATOSCOPY FEATURES

Dermatoscopy discloses additional information to improve the diagnosis (Figures 10.3–10.7).[6–10] MC displays a characteristic pattern composed of a poliglobular white-yellowish amorphous structure in the center of the lesion with a surrounding crown of linear, fine, and sometimes blurred vessels, some of them branching, which do not usually cross the center of the lobules.[6–10] In some cases, curvilinear vessels that form a peripheral reddish ring-like structure that encircles the poliglobular white-yellowish structures can be observed. In more rare cases, arborizing vessels, comma vessels, red globules, and dotted vessels can be seen. Ianhez and colleagues found vascular structures in 89% of the 122 MC of their study. They divided them into three types: crown vessels (72%), radial vessels (54%), and punctiform ("dotted") vessels (20%).[11] They found mixed vascular patterns in 45.7% of lesions.[11]

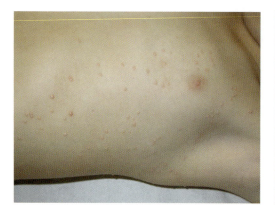

FIGURE 10.1 Several lesions of molluscum contagiosum in a child.

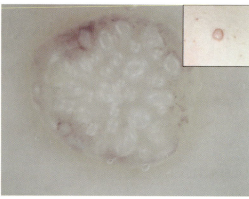

FIGURE 10.4 Dermatoscopy of the typical pattern of molluscum contagiosum.

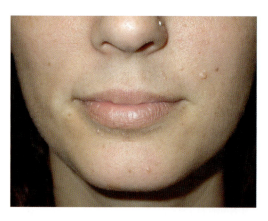

FIGURE 10.2 Lesions of molluscum contagiosum in an adult.

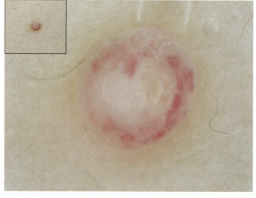

FIGURE 10.5 Dermatoscopy of molluscum contagiosum: central poliglobular white-yellowish amorphous structure surrounded by a peripheral crown of vessels with reddish globules and areas of erythema.

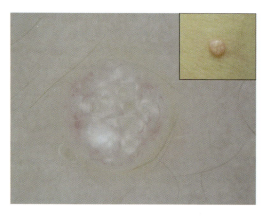

FIGURE 10.3 Dermatoscopy of molluscum contagiosum: central poliglobular white-yellowish amorphous structure and peripheral crown of vessels.

The histopathological correlation of the central poliglobular white-yellowish amorphous structure could be the lobulated, endophytic epidermal hyperplasia with intracytoplasmic inclusion bodies. The crown of vessels or "red corona" corresponds histopathologically to dilated vessels in the dermis that are characteristic of MC. Vázquez-López and colleagues[8] evaluated and classified the dermatoscopic vascular structures seen in 33 nontumoral dermatoses and found this vascular structure in 10 of 15 patients with MC. However, these crown vessels are not solely limited to MC but can be found in sebaceous hyperplasia.[12] In any case, the recognition of this pattern (a central poliglobular white-yellowish amorphous structure surrounded by a peripheral crown of vessels) is very helpful in the clinical diagnosis of MC, especially in adults, helping to differentiate this

Infectious Diseases

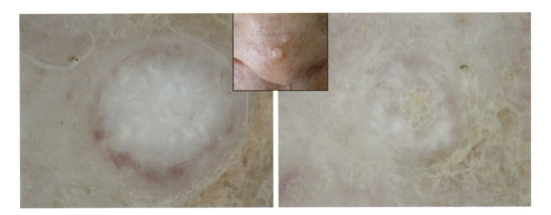

FIGURE 10.6 Two pearly, waxy, dome-shaped papules located on the nose of a 76-year-old man that clinically may resemble basal cell carcinomas. Dermatoscopy of both lesions shows the characteristic pattern of molluscum contagiosum.

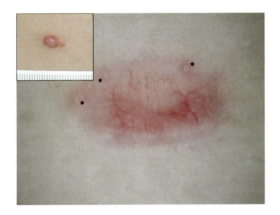

FIGURE 10.7 Dermatoscopy of an atypical case of molluscum contagiosum showing isolated peripheral white-yellowish globules (asterisks) and arborizing vessels throughout the lesion.

infection from many other skin lesions with high confidence. Zaballos and colleagues[7] published an atypical case of a 67-year-old woman with two 5-mm, pearly, waxy, dome-shaped papules of 7-month duration, one located on the thorax and the other on the back, which were clinically diagnosed as basal cell carcinomas and at dermatoscopy as MC because of the characteristic pattern. Histopathology confirmed the diagnosis of MC.

REFERENCES

1. Diven DG. An overview of poxviruses. *J Am Acad Dermatol.* 2001;44:1–14.
2. Brown ST, Nalley JF, Kraus SJ. Molluscum contagiosum. *Sex Transm Dis.* 1981;8:227–34.
3. Hanson D, Diven DG. Molluscum contagiosum. *Dermatol Online J.* 2003;9:2.
4. Gottlieb SL, Myskowki PL. Molluscum contagiosum. *Int J Dermatol.* 1994;33:453–61.
5. Valentine CL, Diven DG, Treatment modalities for molluscum contagiosum. *Dermatol Ther.* 2000;13:285–89.
6. Morales A, Puig S, Zaballos P, Malvehy J. Dermoscopy of Molluscum contagiosum. *Arch Dermatol.* 2005;141:1644.
7. Zaballos P, Ara M, Puig S, Malvehy J. Dermoscopy of molluscum contagiosum: A useful tool for clinical diagnosis in adulthood. *J Eur Acad Dermatol Venereol.* 2006;20:482–83.
8. Vázquez-López F, Kreusch J, Marghoob AA. Dermoscopic semiology: Further insights into vascular features by screening a large spectrum of nontumoral skin lesions. *Br J Dermatol.* 2004;150:226–31.
9. Zalaudek I, Argenziano G, Di Stefani A, et al. Dermoscopy in general dermatology. *Dermatology.* 2006;212:7–18.
10. Zalaudek I, Giacomel J, Cabo H, et al. Entodermoscopy: A new tool for diagnosing skin infections and infestations. *Dermatology.* 2008;216:14–23.
11. Ianhez M, Cestari Sda C, Enokihara MY, Seize MB. Dermoscopic patterns of molluscum contagiosum: A study of 211 lesions confirmed by histopathology. *An Bras Dermatol.* 2011;86:74–79.
12. Zaballos P, Ara M, Puig S, Malvehy J. Dermoscopy of sebaceous hyperplasia. *Arch Dermatol.* 2005;141:808.

11 Infectious diseases
Tinea capitis

Saleh El-Shiemy, Hoda Monieb, Wael Saudi, and Sara Mohy

DEFINITION

Tinea capitis (TC), or scalp ringworm, is a superficial fungal infection of the scalp skin and hair.

EPIDEMIOLOGY/ETIOPATHOGENESIS

TC is a worldwide public health problem that poses specific therapeutic challenges.[1] It is the most common infection of the scalp hair follicles and intervening skin. The epidemiology varies within different geographical areas in the world.[2] TC shows a high incidence in children of tropical countries because warm and humid climate, overcrowded living, and poor sanitary conditions are predisposing factors.[3] Also, direct contact with animals in rural areas should be considered as a potential source of infection.[4] Adult infection occurs infrequently. Several modes of transmission are possible: person-to-person; from affected animals, which represents important asymptomatic carriers; or from soil.[5] Also, TC can be transmitted through hairdressing equipment or in child-care settings.[6] TC is mainly caused by anthropophilic and zoophilic species of the genera *Trichophyton* and *Microsporum*. Three types of hair invasion are recognized: endothrix, ectothrix, or favus.[7]

CLINICAL PRESENTATION/DIAGNOSIS

TC is usually characterized by pruritic, single or multiple patches of alopecia.[8-9] However, it may show different subtypes. It may present with circular alopecic patches showing marked scaling (scaly type) or black dots indicating broken hairs (black dot type), diffuse alopecia with widespread scaling (seborrheic type), boggy nodules studded with pustules (kerion type), and yellow crusts (scutula) that surround hair follicles with a peculiar mousy odor (favus type).[8] TC should be differentiated from seborrheic dermatitis, pityriasis amiantacea, psoriasis, alopecia areata, and trichotillomania; the inflammatory forms should be distinguished from bacterial infections.[10]

Light microscopy of infected hairs and mycological cultures remain the standard criteria for diagnosis of TC.[11]

DERMATOSCOPY/VIDEODERMATOSCOPY FEATURES

As fungal cultures take several days to provide results, dermatoscopy may assist in the initial diagnosis of TC, being particularly useful in detecting early follicular infection when the clinical findings are minimal, in patients with the seborrheic form of TC where the hair loss is often ambiguous,[12] and in dark-skinned patients, in whom erythema of the scalp is difficult to appreciate.[13]

Several features have been described in TC (Figures 11.1–11.8). Slowinska and colleagues in 2008 proposed the "comma hairs" as the distinctive and most prominent dermatoscopic feature of TC by *Microsporum canis* in two Caucasian children, and they considered it as a marker for the diagnosis. Comma hairs were attributed to the cracking and bending of hair shafts filled with the hyphae. It was speculated that this specific type of hairs may represent an intermediate stage in evolution of TC, before formation of dystrophic hairs.[14] A study of seven patients with TC was held by Sandoval and colleagues, who demonstrated the presence of comma hairs in all examined patients. Cultures revealed *Microsporum canis* and *Trichophyton tonsurans*.[15]

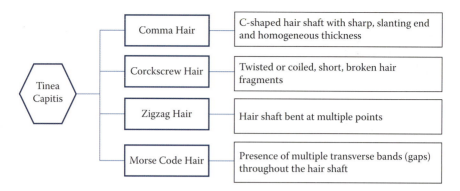

FIGURE 11.1 The main dermatoscopic features of tinea capitis.

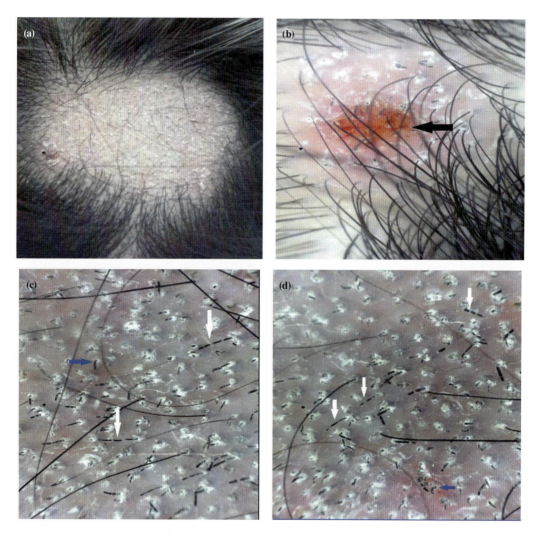

FIGURE 11.2 Scaly type tinea capitis in an 8-year-old male. (a) Clinical aspect. (b–d) Dermatoscopy showing scaling, erythema, and crusts (black arrows), and comma (blue arrows) and Morse code hairs (white arrows) (×10).

Infectious Diseases

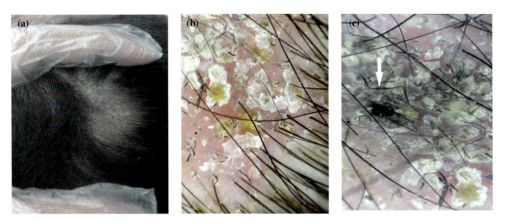

FIGURE 11.3 Scaly type tinea capitis in an 8-year-old female. (a) Clinical aspect. (b–c) Dermatoscopy showing scales (blue arrow), erythema, and zigzag hairs (white arrow) (×10).

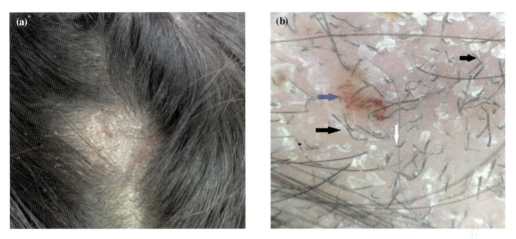

FIGURE 11.4 Scaly type tinea capitis in a 6-year-old female. (a) Clinical aspect. (b) Dermatoscopy revealing scales, erythema, crust (blue arrow), comma hairs (white arrow), and zigzag hairs (black arrows) (×10).

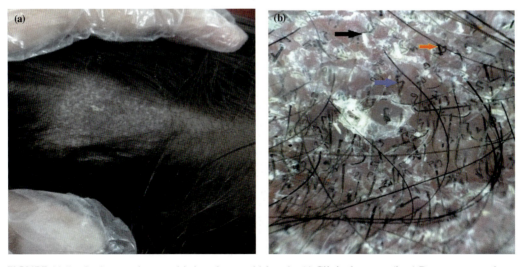

FIGURE 11.5 Scaly type tinea capitis in a 6-year-old female. (a) Clinical aspect. (b–c) Dermatoscopy showing erythema, scales (black arrow), corkscrew (red arrow), and zigzag hairs (blue arrows) (×10).

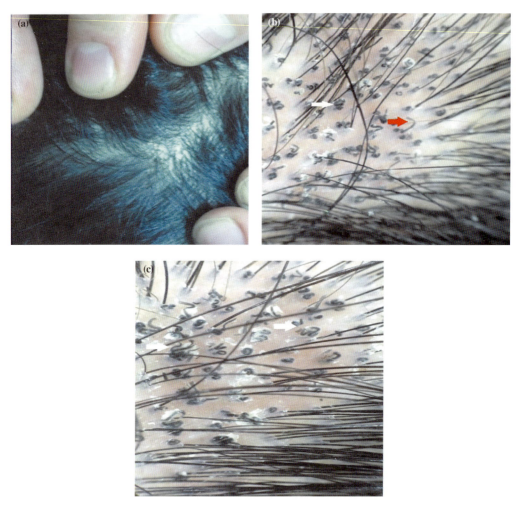

FIGURE 11.6 Black dot–type tinea capitis in a 6-year-old female. (a) Clinical aspect. (b–c) Dermatoscopy showing erythema, comma (red arrow), and corkscrew hairs (white arrows) (×10).

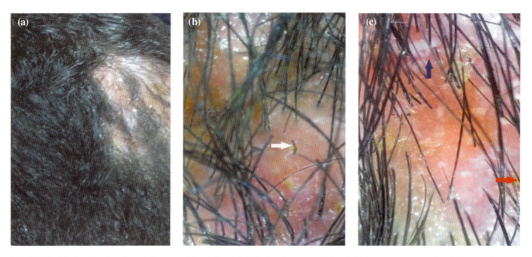

FIGURE 11.7 Kerion in a 6-year-old male. (a) Clinical aspect. (b–c) Dermatoscopy showing erythema, comma hair (white arrow), crusts (red arrow), and pustules (blue arrow) (×10).

Infectious Diseases

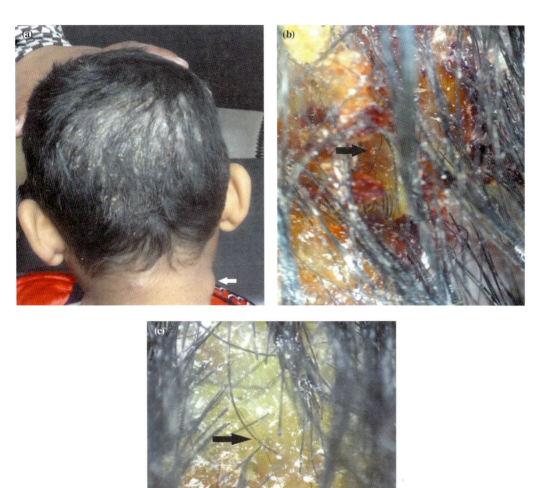

FIGURE 11.8 (a) Favus and enlargement of the posterior cervical lymph nodes (white arrow) in an 8-year-old male. (b–c) Dermatoscopy showing erythema, crusts, and yellow amophorous discharge (black arrow) (×10).

Although comma hairs have been described as a specific dermatoscopic feature of TC, they are not always present. Recognition of additional features is therefore important,[12] and they mainly include corkscrew hairs, zigzag hairs and Morse code hairs. Hughes and colleagues observed corkscrew hairs only in *Tricophyton soudanense* infections,[16] but Vázquez-López and colleagues also detected them in *Tricophyton violaceum* TC.[17] Pinheiro and colleagues concluded that the comma hairs and the corkscrew hairs appear to be specific dermatoscopic findings of dermatophytosis of the scalp, regardless of the etiological agent.[18] However, corkscrew hairs can be seen in patients with ectodermal dysplasias.[19] Zigzag hairs were also described as dermatoscopic feature in TC.[14] They are sharply bent at multiple points and may fracture easily at the bending sites. Zigzag hairs are indicative of TC but also may be seen in other hair and scalp diseases, such as trichorrhexis nodosa, monilethrix, and alopecia areata.[20] Morse code hairs were seen in patients with TC; they are characterized by the presence of multiple transverse bands (gaps) relatively regularly distributed throughout the hair shaft.[19] Finally, other nonspecific trichoscopic findings in TC include broken and dystrophic hairs, i-hair, black dots, and tufted folliculitis.[5]

Rudnicka and colleagues described the dermatoscopic picture of the favus as the presence of yellow scales, big yellow dots lacking hair shafts, large yellowish, wax-colored perifollicular areas, black dots, elongated blood vessels, and, at late stages of the disease, large areas lacking hair. The hair shafts may be normal, slightly curved, or absent. The dermatoscopic findings of kerion were also described by Rudnicka's team as minimal scaling and subtle erythema as well as edematous nodules with or without pustules.[20]

Ultraviolet (UV)-enhanced trichoscopy, first described in 2011 by Rudnicka and colleagues, is a new method that may help identify TC. It is based on dermatoscopy, but regular light is replaced by UV light at a wavelength overlapping or partly overlapping Wood's light.[19]

In 2014, in a series of 70 Egyptian children (unpublished data), the scaly type of TC was the predominant presentation (23.9%) followed by black dot type. The dermatoscopic findings for TC showed that scales were present in 93.5% of cases, erythema in 79.2%, and crusts in 57.1%. The characteristic findings of TC were comma hairs in 46.7% of the cases, corkscrew hairs in 38.9%, zigzag hairs in 18.1%, and Morse code hairs in 11.6% of cases; i-hairs and hair casts had the same percentage each (7.8%), while yellow amophorous discharge was seen only in favus cases, with the percentage of 3.8%.

Dermatoscopy may help in the differential diagnosis with other scalp disorders that may present similar clinical features but show different dermatoscopic findings: seborrheic dermatitis shows yellowish scale, arborizing vessels, and atypical red vessels;[19] psoriasis shows areas of thick silvery-white scaling with interfollicular twisted red loops;[21] pityriasis amiantacea shows yellowish concretions that form thick, matted bundles holding the hairs together;[22] alopecia areata shows yellow dots, black dots, tapering hairs (exclamation mark and coudability hairs), circle hairs, and hypopigmented vellus hairs;[15] trichotillomania shows breakage of hair at different lengths, short hairs with trichoptilosis, irregular coiled hairs, amorphous hair residues, black dots, micro–exclamation mark, flame Hairs, V-sign, hook hairs, hair powder, and tulip hairs.[23]

Note from the Editors: High magnification VD (×150) of TC caused by *Microsporum canis* has revealed additional features not visible at low magnifications: horizontal white bands, bent hairs, broken hairs, and translucent, easily deformable hairs (Figure 11.9).[24] They may be explained as follows: the horizontal white bands, observed at low magnification in the so-called Morse code hairs, at higher magnification appear as "empty" bands likely related to localized areas of fungal infection; they are usually multiple and represent *loci minoris resistentiae* that may cause the hairs to eventually bend (bent hairs), configuring the zigzag hairs, and break (broken hairs). Translucent, easily deformable hairs may be sometimes observed and look weakened and transparent, showing unusual bends; they are likely the result of a massive fungal invasion involving the whole hair shaft.[24]

REFERENCES

1. Ali J, Yifru S, Woldeamanuel Y. Prevalence of tinea capitis and the causative agent among school children in Gondar, North West Ethiopia. *Ethiop Med.* 2009;47:261–69.
2. Mebazaa, E. Oumari K, N. Ghariani, et al. Tinea capitis in adults in Tunisia. *Int J Dermatol.* 2010;49:513–16.
3. Sajjan G, Mangalgi S. Clinicomycological profile of tinea capitis in children residing in orphanages. *Int J Biol Med Res.* 2012;3:2405–07.
4. Azab M, Mahmoud N, Abd Allah S, et al. Dermatophytes isolated from clinical samples of children suffering from tinea capitis in Ismailia, Egypt. *Aust. J. Basic & Appl. Sci.* 2011;6:38–42.
5. Cervetti O, Albini P, Arese V, et al. Tinea capitis in adults. *Adv Microbiol.* 2014;4:12–14.
6. El-Khalawany M, Shaaban D, Hassan H, et al. A multicenter clinicomycological study evaluating the spectrum of adult tinea capitis in Egypt. *Acta Dermatovenerol Alp Panonica Adriat.* 2013;22:77–82.

Infectious Diseases

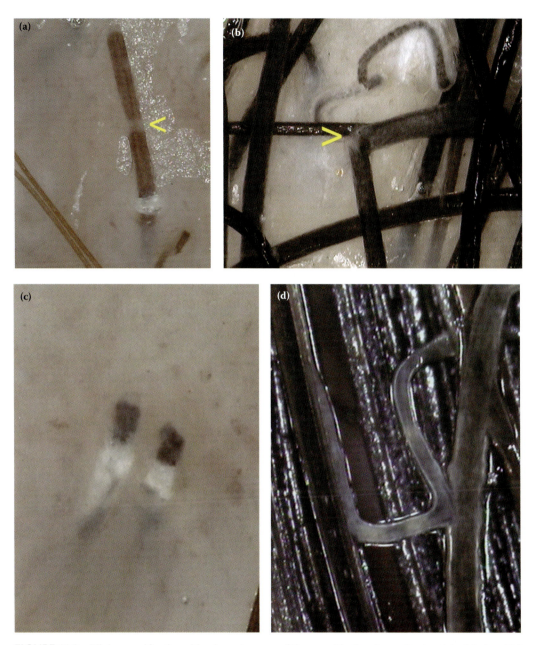

FIGURE 11.9 High-magnification videodermatoscopy of tinea capitis showing an horizontal white band (a), bent hairs (b), broken hairs. (c), and translucent, easily deformable hairs (d) (×150).

7. Kakourou T, Uksal U. Guidelines for the management of tinea capitis in children. *Pediatr Dermatol*. 2010;27:226–28.
8. Seebacher C, Bouchara JP, Mignon B. Updates on the epidemiology of dermatophyte infections. *Mycopathologia*. 2008;166:335–52.
9. Trovato MJ, Schwartz RA, Janniger CK. Tinea capitis: Current concepts in clinical practice. *Cutis*. 2006;77:93–99.
10. Ilkit M and Demirhindi H. Asymptomatic dermatophyte scalp carriage: Laboratory diagnosis, epidemiology and management. *Mycopathologia*. 2008;165:61–71.
11. Haliasos EC, Kerner M, Jaimes-Lopez N, et al. Dermoscopy for the pediatric dermatologist part I: Dermoscopy of pediatric infectious and inflammatory skin lesions and hair disorders. *Pediatr Dermatol*. 2013;30:163–71.

12. Lin YT, Li YC. The dermoscopic comma, zigzag, and bar code-like hairs: Markers of fungal infection of the hair follicles. *Dermatol Sinica.* 2014;32:160–63.
13. Mapelli ET, Gualandri L, Cerri A, Menni S. Comma hairs in tinea capitis: A useful dermatoscopic sign for diagnosis of tinea capitis. *Pediatr Dermatol.* 2012;29:223–24.
14. Slowinska M, Rudnicka L, Schwartz RA, et al. Comma hairs: A dermatoscopic marker for tinea capitis: A rapid diagnostic method *J Am Acad Dermatol.* 2008;59:S77–79.
15. Sandoval AB, Ortiz JA, Rodriguez JM, et al. Dermoscopic pattern in tinea capitis. *Rev Iberoam Micol.* 2010;27:151–52.
16. Hughes R, Chiaverini C, Bahadoran P, Lacour JP. Corkscrew hair: A new dermoscopic sign for diagnosis of tinea capitis in black children. *Arch Dermatol.* 2011;147:355–56.
17. Vázquez-López F, Palacios-Garcia L, Argenziano G. Dermoscopic corkscrew hairs dissolve after successful therapy of Trichophyton violaceum tinea capitis: A case report. *Australas J Dermatol.* 2012;53:118–19.
18. Pinheiro AMC, Lobato LA, Varella TCN. Dermoscopy findings in tinea capitis. Case report and literature review. *An Bras Dermatol.* 2012;8:313–14.
19. Rudnicka L, Olszewska M, Rakowska A, et al. Trichoscopy update. *J Dermatol Case Rep.* 2011;4:82–88.
20. Rudnicka L. Olszewska M, Rakowska A (eds.). *Atlas of Trichoscopy.* London: Springer-Verlag, 2012.
21. Kim G, Jung H, Ko H, et al. Dermoscopy can be useful in differentiating scalp psoriasis from seborrhoeic dermatitis. *Br J Dermatol.* 2011;164:652–56.
22. Rogers N. Scoping scalp disorders: Practical use of a novel dermatoscope to diagnose hair and scalp conditions. *J Drugs Dermatol.* 2013;12:283–86.
23. Rakowska A, Slowinska M, Olszewska M, et al. New trichoscopy findings in trichotillomania: Flame hairs, V-sign, hook hairs, hair powder, tulip hairs. *Acta Derm Venereol.* 2014;94:303–6.
24. Lacarrubba F, Verzì AE, Micali G. Newly described features resulting from high-magnification dermatoscopy of tinea capitis. *JAMA Dermatol.* 2015;151(3):308–10.

12 Hair loss and hair shaft disorders

Antonella Tosti

Dermoscopy is a very useful and fast tool for diagnosis of hair and scalp disorders, including hair shaft disorders.[1-6] For scalp examination, dermatologists may use a manual dermatoscope (×10 magnification) or a videodermatoscope equipped with various lenses (from ×20–×1000 magnification). Both epiluminescent and non-epiluminescent modes are employed, and alcohol or thermal water can be used as interface solutions.

Dermoscopy findings in hair and scalp disorders include follicular and interfollicular patterns, as well as the hair shaft's characteristics (Table 12.1).

NORMAL SCALP

Examination of the normal scalp shows a diffuse white color and often simple fine red loops, which represent capillary loops in the dermal papilla. Follicular units contain 2–3 terminal hairs and 1 or 2 vellus hairs (Figure 12.1). In dark-skinned individuals (phototypes V and VI), a perifollicular pigmented network (honeycomb pattern) is well appreciated. The network consists of hyperchromic lines that represent melanocytes in the rete ridge system in contrast with hypochromic areas formed by fewer melanocytes localized in the supra papillary epidermis. Small white dots, or pinpoint white dots, are regularly distributed among follicular units (Figure 12.2).

ANDROGENETIC ALOPECIA

AGA is the most common form of hair loss, affecting up to 80% of men and 50% of women. Patients typically present with progressive thinning and shortening of hair in androgen-dependent scalp regions including frontal, temporal, and vertex areas.

DERMOSCOPIC FEATURES

Hair diameter diversity

In general, scalp examination in AGA should be taken in an area delineated at the cross between the nose line and the ear implantation line.

The progressive miniaturization of hair with visualization of hairs with different calibers is enhanced by dermoscopic examination. A hair diameter diversity of >20% is diagnostic of AGA and is significantly correlated to follicle miniaturization by histological analysis (Figure 12.3).[7] It is worthwhile to note that follicular ostia in AGA show predominance of single hairs, instead of 2–4 hair shafts observed in normal subjects. Presence of more than 10% or 7 short vellus hair at ×20 magnification at the frontal hairline is diagnostic for AGA in women (Figure 12.4).[8]

Other features of AGA include peripilar brown halos at the follicular ostia, seen in patients with early AGA, yellow dots in patients with severe AGA (Figure 12.3), and honeycomb-like pigmented network on sun-exposed scalp.

ALOPECIA AREATA

Alopecia areata is an autoimmune, nonscarring form of alopecia. A wide range of clinical presentations can occur, from single patch of alopecia to complete loss of scalp hair (alopecia totalis) or hair of the entire body (alopecia universalis). The disease affects most commonly scalp hairs, but it may also involve eyebrows, eyelashes, beard, pubic, axillary, and all body hairs.

TABLE 12.1
Dermoscopic patterns in normal and pathological scalp

Interfollicular patterns
- Vascular patterns
  - Simple red loops
  - Twisted red loops
  - Arborizing red lines
  - Red dots
- Pigment pattern: honeycomb pigmented network
- Blue-gray dots

Follicular patterns
- Yellow dots
- Red dots
- Peripilar sign
- Pinpoint white dots
- Keratotic plugs
- Black dots

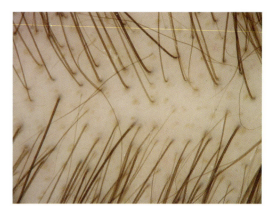

FIGURE 12.3 Dermoscopy of androgenetic alopecia: hair shaft variability and yellow dots (×20).

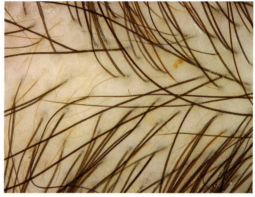

FIGURE 12.4 Dermoscopy of androgenetic alopecia: presence of more than 7 thin, short vellus hairs (20×).

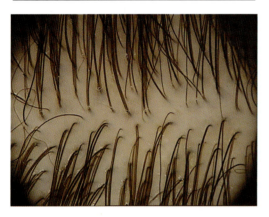

FIGURE 12.1 Dermoscopy of normal scalp of a Caucasian patient: diffuse white color and follicular units containing 1–3 terminal hairs (×20).

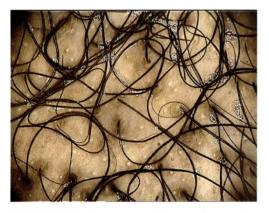

FIGURE 12.2 Dermoscopy of black scalp: pinpoint white dots in the interfollicular scalp (×20).

DERMOSCOPIC FEATURES

Yellow dots

The presence of yellow dots is a characteristic finding in alopecia areata. This pattern is characterized by a distinctive array of yellow to yellow-red, round and polycyclic dots that vary in size and correspond to the dilated follicular openings with or without hair shafts (Figure 12.5). Yellow dots are seen in Caucasian and Asian patients but not in patients with dark scalp, where the hair follicles appear as pinpoint white dots (Figure 12.6).

Dystrophic hairs

Dystrophic hair shafts are well appreciated by dermoscopy even at lower magnification (×10). In active alopecia areata, the anagen arrest causes hair shafts to fracture before emergence

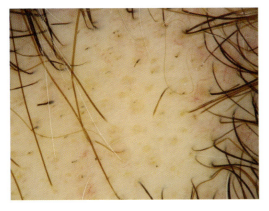

FIGURE 12.5 Dermoscopy of alopecia areata: yellow dots and broken dystrophic hairs (×20).

from the scalp: these cadaverized hairs appear as black dots at dermoscopy (Figures 12.5–12.7). Growing of the broken shafts leads to formation of exclamation mark hairs, which are characterized by a distal irregular fractured tip that is darker and wider than the proximal portion of the shaft (Figure 12.8).

Other features seen in alopecia areata include pseudo-monilethrix, due to variation in the caliber of the hairs shaft; short regrowing, miniaturized, and vellus hairs (shorter than 10 mm); and circle hairs (Figure 12.9).

Dermoscopy is useful for assessing disease activity and prognosis (Figure 12.10).

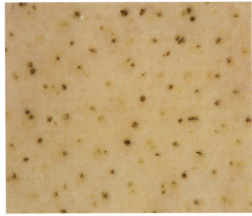

FIGURE 12.7 Dermoscopy of alopecia areata: black dots (×20).

ALOPECIA AREATA INCOGNITA

Alopecia areata incognita was first described by Rebora in 1987, and is characterized by acute onset of diffuse shedding of telogen hairs in the absence of typical patches. Patients are often concerned about severe thinning within a few months. Differential diagnosis with AGA and telogen effluvium is often difficult, and dermoscopy has proved to be an important tool in this challenging diagnosis.[9]

FIGURE 12.6 Dermoscopy of alopecia areata totalis in a dark-skinned patient: follicular openings appear as pinpoint white dots (×20).

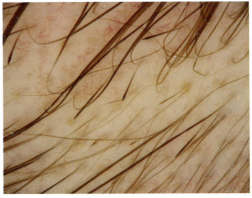

FIGURE 12.8 Dermoscopy of alopecia areata: exclamation mark hairs (×20).

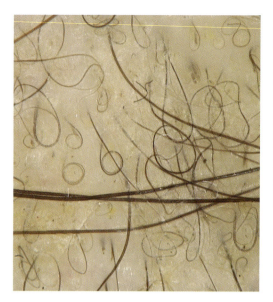

FIGURE 12.9 Dermoscopy of alopecia areata: circle hairs (×20).

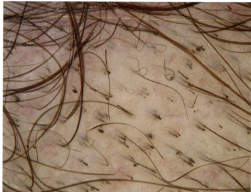

FIGURE 12.10 Dermoscopy of active alopecia areata: black dots and broken hairs (×20).

DERMOSCOPIC FEATURES

Presence of yellow dots and short regrowing hairs suggests diagnosis. Exclamation mark hairs and cadaverized hairs are not common.

TRICHOTILLOMANIA

Trichotillomania is a compulsive disorder in which individuals pull out hair from the scalp or any other body area, resulting in alopecic patches. It is relatively more common in children.

On physical exam, irregular patches of hair loss, with typical bizarre borders, are observed. Inside the plaques, short broken hairs with variable lengths are evident.

Dermoscopic features may be difficult to distinguish from alopecia areata. These include yellow dots, question mark hairs characterized by a coiled tip, black dots, flame hairs, broken hair shafts with different lengths, and longitudinal splitting of the hair shafts (Figure 12.10).

CONGENITAL TRIANGULAR ALOPECIA

Congenital triangular alopecia usually presents in children between 3 and 6 years as a triangular or oval patch of alopecia most frequently localized in the fronto-temporal hairline. Dermoscopy is helpful in the diagnosis when the triangular alopecia has an atypical location. Dermoscopy of the patch shows normal follicular openings and a carpet of vellus hairs surrounded by normal terminal hairs in the adjacent scalp.[10,11]

SCARRING ALOPECIA

Cicatricial alopecias include a group of hair disorders that cause permanent destruction of the hair follicles. Causes of cicatricial alopecias are categorized as primary or secondary. Primary cicatricial alopecias specifically target the hair follicle and result in its destruction. In secondary scarring alopecias, the hair follicle destruction is secondary to diffuse scarring of the dermis.

Differential diagnosis of cicatricial alopecias requires a scalp biopsy. Dermoscopy has shown to be useful for finding appropriate sites from which to take biopsies, as well as to provide new information about the diseases. In all types of cicatricial alopecias, scalp examination reveals variable degrees of absence of follicular ostia.

LICHEN PLANOPILARIS

Lichen planopilaris (LPP) is the most common cause of cicatricial alopecia and affects middle-aged women most frequently. Patients present

Hair Loss and Hair Shaft Disorders

with scalp itching and tenderness. Scalp examination shows irregular patches of hair loss, which become confluent, affecting most frequently the parietal and vertex regions. The disease has a progressive course, and severe alopecia may develop in some patients.

Dermoscopic features

Dermoscopy reveals absence of follicular openings and peripilar casts around the hairs at the periphery of the patch (Figures 12.11–12.12). Round perifollicular blue-gray dots with a "target pattern" can be observed in some dark patients with LPP. This pattern is due to the presence of melanophages around hair follicles, sparing interfollicular epidermis.

In frontal fibrosing alopecia, a clinical variant of lichen planopilaris, the most prominent dermoscopic findings are loss of follicular openings, loss of vellus hairs, peripilar scales, and peripilar erythema (Figures 12.13–12.14).[12]

DISCOID LUPUS ERYTHEMATOSUS

Discoid lupus erythematosus (DLE) of the scalp is characterized by single or multiple alopecic patches. Affected scalp shows erythema, scaling, follicular plugging, atrophy and telangiectasias. Despite the fact that is considered as part of the group of cicatricial alopecias, DLE often shows hair regrowth if promptly treated. In this way, early diagnosis is important for patients' prognosis.

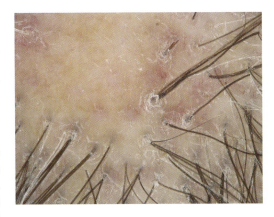

FIGURE 12.12 Dermoscopy of lichen planopilaris: loss of follicular openings, scalp erythema, and peripilar casts (×20).

Dermoscopic features

Scalp atrophy is represented by a diffuse white color of the scalp. This pattern is well appreciated in dark-skinned patients, who lose the normally seen pigmented network within the lesion. The honeycomb pigmented network might be seen at the periphery of the plaque of DLE.

Arborizing and tortuous vessels are the most common vascular patterns seen inside DLE plaques (Figure 12.15). Hyperkeratotic follicular pluggings are a very common finding

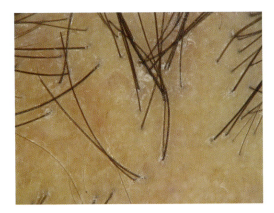

FIGURE 12.11 Dermoscopy of lichen planopilaris: loss of follicular openings and presence of peripilar casts (×20).

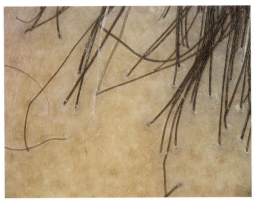

FIGURE 12.13 Dermoscopy of frontal fibrosing alopecia: absence of vellus hairs and presence of peripilar casts (×20).

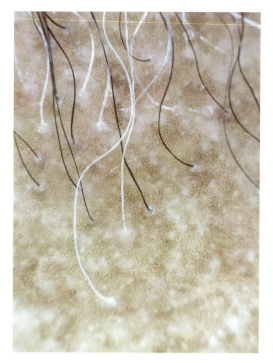

FIGURE 12.14 Dermoscopy of frontal fibrosing alopecia in a dark-skinned patient: absence of vellus hairs, peripilar casts irregular distributed, pinpoint white dots, and irregular white patches (×20).

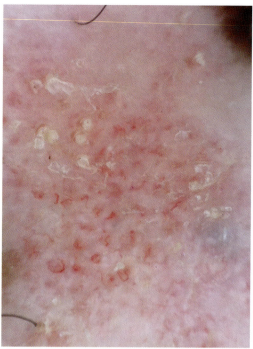

FIGURE 12.15 Dermoscopy of discoid lupus erythematosus: enlarged branching vessels, loss of pigment, and keratotic plugs (×20).

(Figure 12.15).[13] The presence of red dots has been associated with good prognosis with hair regrowth after treatment (Figure 12.16). Blue-gray dots may be observed with a diffuse and speckled pattern of distribution, as pigmental incontinence affects the papillary dermis of the follicular and interfollicular epidermis.

Folliculitis decalvans

Folliculitis decalvans (FD) is a neutrophilic variant of cicatricial alopecias, which accounts for approximately 11% of all primary cicatricial alopecias. FD usually starts with follicular papules and pustules on the vertex and/or occipital area of the scalp, followed by intense inflammatory reaction and development of an indurated and boggy scarring patch. Multiple hair tufts are often found emerging from a common dilated follicular opening. *S. aureus* can be isolated from FD lesions and seems to play an important role in the inflammatory process.

Dermoscopic features

Dermoscopy shows severe scaling and crusting, and tufted hair shafts (Figure 12.17). Presence of tufts of more than 6 hairs emerging together and surrounded by concentric scales suggests a diagnosis (Figure 12.18). Multiple coiled dilated capillary loops, similar to those observed in psoriasis, and arborizing red lines are typical findings seen all over the affected scalp (Figure 12.19).

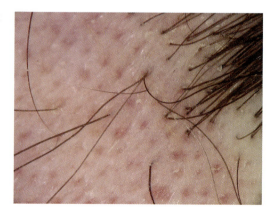

FIGURE 12.16 Dermoscopy of discoid lupus erythematosus: red dot pattern (×20).

Hair Loss and Hair Shaft Disorders

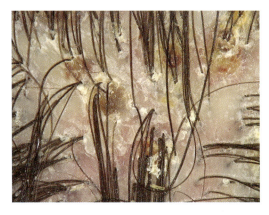

FIGURE 12.17 Dermoscopy of folliculitis decalvans: scalp scaling with hemorrhagic crusts (×20).

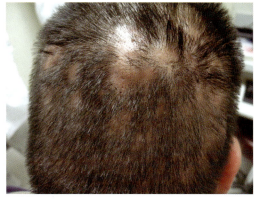

FIGURE 12.20 Dissecant cellulitis: alopecic patches overlying nodular scalp lesions.

Dissecting cellulitis of the scalp

Dissecting cellulitis is a rare disorder seen mostly in young males of Afro-American descent. The scalp presents patches of alopecia overlying painful suppurative nodules and fluctuating abscesses (Figure 12.20).

Dermoscopic features

Dermoscopy shows a pattern of non-scarring alopecia, enlarged plugged follicular openings, black dots and broken hairs[14] (Figure 12.21).

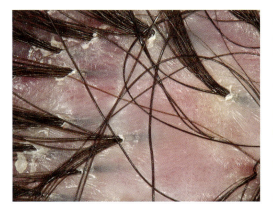

FIGURE 12.18 Dermoscopy of folliculitis decalvans: tuft of hairs emerging together surrounded by concentric scales (×20).

Central centrifugal cicatricial alopecia

Central centrifugal cicatricial alopecia (CCCA) is a common scarring alopecia affecting women of African descent. The alopecia affects the top of the scalp and spread centrifugally (Figure 12.22).

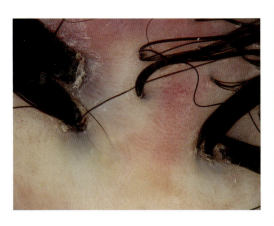

FIGURE 12.19 Dermoscopy of folliculitis decalvans: coiled vessels and hair tufting (×20).

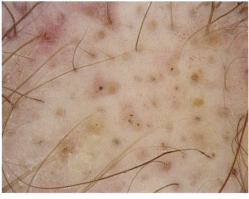

FIGURE 12.21 Dermoscopy of dissecant cellulitis in a Caucasian patient: nonscarring alopecia with yellow dots and black dots (×20).

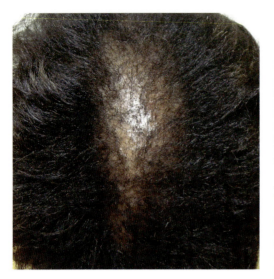

FIGURE 12.22 Central centrifugal cicatricial alopecia: alopecia of the central scalp.

Dermoscopic features

Dermoscopy shows a preserved honeycomb pattern, pinpoint white dots with irregular distribution, and irregular white patches, corresponding to follicular scarring. The presence of a peripilar gray-white halo around the preserved hairs within the patch highly suggests diagnosis (Figure 12.23). Broken hairs and black dots can occasionally be seen.[15]

Traction alopecia

Traction alopecia is extremely common in women and children of African descent, in whom it affects the marginal scalp, particularly the frontal and the temporal scalp. In the early phase, the alopecia is reversible but it becomes permanent in longstanding disease. The bald patch typically mantains some vellus hairs and presents a rim of preserved hairs at the hairline (Figure 12.24).

Dermoscopic features

Dermoscopy shows irregular pinpoint white dots, vellus hairs, broken hairs and black dots. Presence of hair casts around the hair at the periphery of the patches indicates that the patient's hairstyle is still causing traction (Figure 12.25).[16]

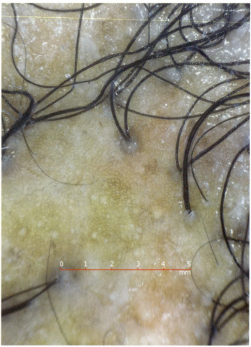

FIGURE 12.23 Dermoscopy of central centrifugal cicatricial alopecia: gray-white halos surrounding the emerging hairs (×20).

HAIR SHAFT DISORDERS

The most important advantage of dermoscopy in the evaluation of hair shaft disorders is that

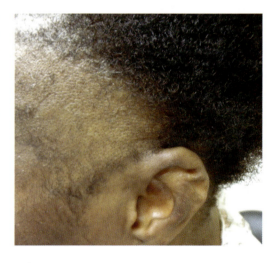

FIGURE 12.24 Traction alopecia: "fringe sign."

Hair Loss and Hair Shaft Disorders

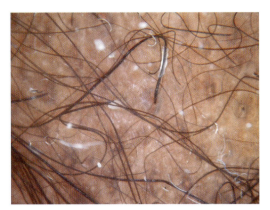

FIGURE 12.25 Dermoscopy of traction alopecia: hair casts surrounding the hair shaft at the periphery of the patch (×40).

it is painless and allows for screening the entire scalp along with the eyebrows and eyelashes that may be the only affected site in some conditions. This is of great importance as most of these disorders are seen in children.[17]

Hair shaft disorders associated with increased fragility

Monilethrix

Monilethrix is an autosomal dominant disorder, with variable expression, due to mutations of the human basic hair keratins hHb6 and hHb1. The hair is dull, fragile, and breaks easily, especially in the sites of friction such as the nape and occipital areas. Follicular keratosis of the affected scalp and keratosis pilaris are also typical. (Figure 12.26).

Dermoscopy reveals typical beading, characterized by elliptical nodes and intermittent constrictions at regular distance (Figure 12.27). Breakage occurs at constriction level and broken hairs bend in different directions (Figure 12.28).

Trichorrhexis invaginata

Trichorrhexis invaginata is a very rare hair shaft disorder that characterizes Netherton disease, an autosomal recessive genodermatosis which combines ichthyosis, trichorrhexis invaginata and atopic dermatitis. Hair fragility and breakage cause alopecia, which is more severe in scalp areas exposed to friction; it frequently affects eyelashes and eyebrows that may present the abnormality even when the scalp hair, which improves with age, appears normal.

In trichorrhexis invaginata the hair shaft is similar to a bamboo shoot due to the presence of multiple knots along its length. Breakage occurs in correspondence with the knots.

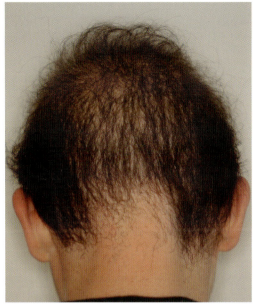

FIGURE 12.26 Monilethrix: alopecia due to hair breakage more evident on the nape.

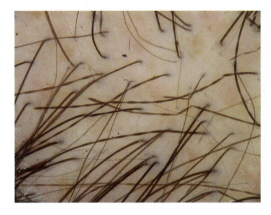

FIGURE 12.27 Dermoscopy of monilethrix: hair beading and breakage (×20).

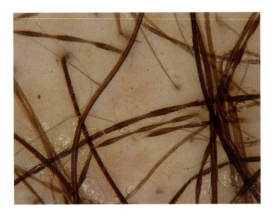

FIGURE 12.28 Dermoscopy of monilethrix: breakage occurs at internode levels (×40).

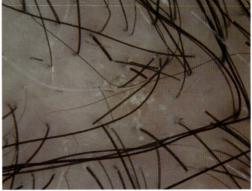

FIGURE 12.29 Dermoscopy of trichorrhexis nodosa: proximal lesions of hair shafts caused by scratching (×20).

Dermoscopy shows nodular swellings at irregular intervals. The ball-shaped knots are similar to matchsticks. The broken shafts often have a ragged, cupped shape.

Trichorrhexis nodosa

Trichorrhexis nodosa is a very common acquired hair shaft disorder that causes hair breakage. It mostly affects the distal part of long damaged hairs. Causes of trichorrhexis nodosa include mechanical, physical and chemical procedures that damage the hair shaft.

Proximal trichorrhexis nodosa can be a consequence of intense scratching (Figure 12.29).

At dermoscopy the hair shaft shows multiple swollen white areas that correspond to the sites of future fracturing. At higher magnification they appear as the ends of two brushes aligned in opposition (Figure 12.30). Fractured shafts appear as paintbrushes (Figure 12.31).

Pili torti

Pili torti are a feature of some rare syndromes, including Menkes syndrome. Isolated pili torti, however, are not diagnostic, as they are often seen in patients with cicatricial alopecia, particularly lichen planopilaris and frontal fibrosing alopecia (Figure 12.32). They are also seen in ectodermal dysplasias or in association with other hair shaft abnormalities.

Dermoscopy shows a flattened hair shaft with irregular twistings (Figure 12.33).

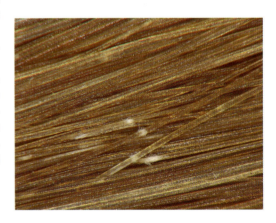

FIGURE 12.30 Dermoscopy of trichorrhexis nodosa: the hair shafts show multiple white areas with fibrillar destruction (×40).

Hair Loss and Hair Shaft Disorders

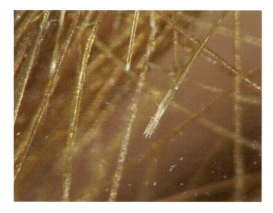

FIGURE 12.31 Dermoscopy of trichorrhexis nodosa: brush-like stumps (×50).

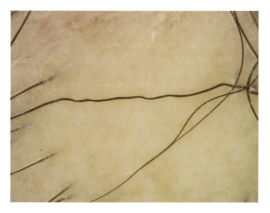

FIGURE 12.32 Dermoscopy of pili torti in a patient with scarring alopecia (×20).

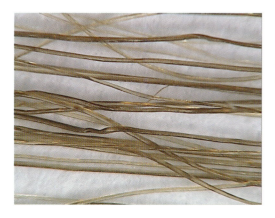

FIGURE 12.33 Dermoscopy of pili torti: irregular twisting of the hair shaft (×20).

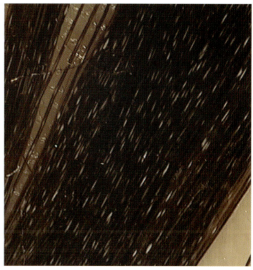

FIGURE 12.34 Dermoscopy of pili annulati: the hair shafts present regular white bands (×20).

Pili annulati

Pili annulati is an autosomal dominant hair shaft abnormality, which is more commonly diagnosed incidentally, as it does not cause alopecia or hair fragility. The hair often looks very beautiful as has a shiny appearance.

Dermoscopy shows regularly distributed white bands that correspond to air-filled cavities within the hair cortex (Figure 12.34).

Pili trianguli and canaliculi

Pili trianguli and canaliculi can be autosomal dominant or sporadic. The hair shaft abnormality causes uncombable hair that look dry, spun-glass, and unruly. The condition improves spontaneously with ageing.

Dermoscopy shows that the hair shaft has a triangular or reniform shape with a longitudinal groove (Figure 12.35).

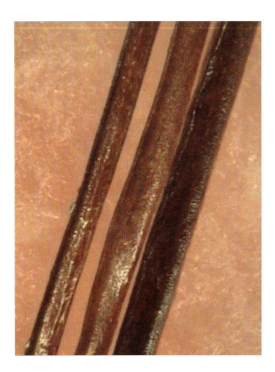

FIGURE 12.35 Dermoscopy of pili trianguli and canaliculi: longitudinal groove of the hair shaft (×40).

REFERENCES

1. Ross EK, Vincenzi C, Tosti A. Videodermoscopy in the evaluation of hair and scalp disorders. *J Am Acad Dermatol.* 2006;55:799–806.
2. Lacarruba F, Dall'Oglio F, Nasca MR, Micali G. Videodermatoscopy enhances diagnostic capability in some forms of hair loss. *Am J Clin Dermatol.* 2004;5:205–8.
3. Torres F, Tosti A. Trichoscopy: An update. *G Ital Dermatol Venereol.* 2014;149(1):83–91.
4. Miteva M, Tosti A. Hair and scalp dermatoscopy. *J Am Acad Dermatol.* 2012;67(5):1040–8.
5. Lencastre A, Tosti A. Role of trichoscopy in children's scalp and hair disorders. *Pediatr Dermatol.* 2013;30(6):674–82.
6. Torres F, Tosti A. Trichoscopy: An update. *G Ital Dermatol Venereol.* 2014;149(1):83–91.
7. de Lacharrière O, Deloche C, Misciali C, et al. Hair diameter diversity: A clinical sign reflecting the follicle miniaturization. *Arch Dermatol.* 2001;137:641–46.
8. Herskovitz I, de Sousa IC, Tosti A. Vellus hairs in the frontal scalp in early female pattern hair loss. *Int J Trichology.* 2013;5(3):118–20.
9. Tosti A, Whiting D, Iorizzo M, et al. The role of scalp dermoscopy in the diagnosis of alopecia areata incognita. *J Am Acad Dermatol.* 2008;59:64–67.
10. Iorizzo M, Pazzaglia M, Starace M, et al. Videodermoscopy: A useful tool for diagnosing congenital triangular alopecia. *Pediatr Dermatol.* 2008;25(6):652–54.
11. Lacarrubba F, Micali G. Congenital triangular alopecia. *BMJ Case Rep.* 2014;2014.
12. Lacarrubba F, Micali G, Tosti A. Absence of vellus hair in the hairline: A videodermatoscopic feature of frontal fibrosing alopecia. *Br J Dermatol.* 2013;169(2):473.
13. Lanuti E, Miteva M, Romanelli P, Tosti A. Trichoscopy and histopathology of follicular keratotic plugs in scalp discoid lupus erythematosus. *Int J Trichology.* 2012;4(1):36–38.
14. Tosti A, Torres F, Miteva M. Dermoscopy of early dissecting cellulitis of the scalp simulates alopecia areata. *Actas Dermosifiliogr.* 2013;104(1):92–93.
15. Miteva M, Tosti A. Dermatoscopic features of central centrifugal cicatricial alopecia. *J Am Acad Dermatol.* 2014;71(3):443–49.
16. Yin NC, Tosti A. A systematic approach to Afro-textured hair disorders: Dermatoscopy and when to biopsy. *Dermatol Clin.* 2014;32(2):145–51.
17. Miteva M, Tosti A. Dermatoscopy of hair shaft disorders. *J Am Acad Dermatol.* 2013;68(3):473–81.

13 Inflammatory diseases
Psoriasis

Francesco Lacarrubba, Giorgio Filosa, Rossella De Angelis, Leonardo Bugatti, Maria Concetta Potenza, Ilaria Proietti, Robert A. Schwartz, Maria Letizia Musumeci, Maria Rita Nasca, Paolo Rosina, and Giuseppe Micali

DEFINITION

Psoriasis is a common, chronic, relapsing, inflammatory skin disorder with genetic predisposition, multifactorial pathogenesis, and variable morphology, distribution, and severity. It is characterized by abnormal keratinocytic hyperproliferation resulting in thickening of the epidermis and stratum corneum.

EPIDEMIOLOGY/ETIOPATHOGENESIS

Psoriasis affects about 3% of the overall population of the world.[1] The most common variant is psoriasis vulgaris or plaque-type. Psoriasis develops as a result of abnormal keratinocytes proliferation and differentiation, associated with local activation of the Th1/Th17-type response and with vascular modifications.

CLINICAL PRESENTATION/DIAGNOSIS

Plaque-type psoriasis is characterized by sharply demarcated, well-circumscribed reddish and scaly plaques more often located on the elbows, knees and scalp. Other body areas, as well as the nails, may also be affected.[1-2] Other variants include palmo-plantar psoriasis, inverse psoriasis, and psoriatic balanitis.

Histopathologically, psoriasis is the prototype of a group of cutaneous disorders that shows psoriasiform epidermal hyperplasia (psoriasiform dermatitis), defined as regular elongation of the rete ridges.[3] Three main phases may be observed: the *initial phase*, the *intermediate or steady-state phase* (divided into *early* and *late steady-state*), and the *phase of resolution*. The initial phase can be not specific, with a preponderance of dermal changes, including a sparse superficial perivascular T-lymphocytic infiltrate (Figure 13.1). The early steady-state phase, that clinically corresponds to the presence of erythematous edematous plaques, is characterized by acanthosis with regular elongation of the rete ridges, thickening in their lower portion, thinning of the suprapapillary epidermis with occasional presence of small spongiform pustules, diminished to absent granular layer, confluent parakeratosis, and presence of Munro microabscesses (Figure 13.2). It is possible to find elongation and edema of the dermal papillae, and dilated and tortuous capillaries. Although elongation of the dermal papillary vessels is not exclusive to psoriasis, the striking difference in psoriasis is that these changes are dramatic and uniformly distributed throughout the clinical lesions.[4] The combination of superficial dermal capillaries and overlying suprapapillary epidermal thinning is responsible for the erythematous appearance of psoriatic lesion and the Auspitz's sign (pinpoint bleeding points on removal of the scale). The late steady-state phase, which clinically corresponds to classical plaques, is characterized by club-shaped thickening of the lower rete pegs with coalescence of these in some areas. Lesions show silvery scales as result of the orthokeratosis of corneum and an intact granular layer with parakeratosis. Exocytosis of inflammatory cells is usually mild and there is some thickening of the suprapapillary plates and fine fibrillary collagen (Figure 13.3). The phase of resolution corresponds to resolving

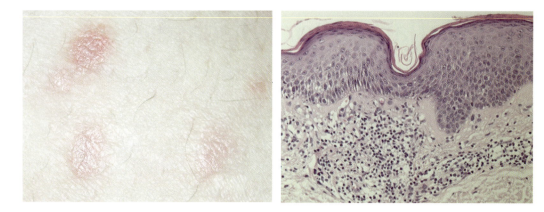

FIGURE 13.1 Plaque psoriasis: clinical and histological features of the initial phase.

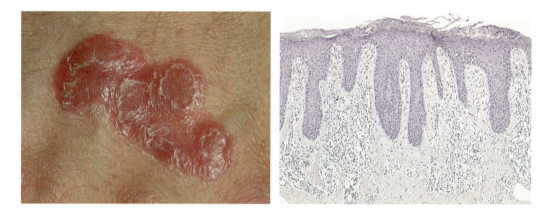

FIGURE 13.2 Plaque psoriasis: clinical and histological features of the early steady-state phase.

or treated plaques of psoriasis (Figure 13.4). It initially shows progressive reduction of neutrophils within the stratum corneum and parakeratosis, with reconstruction of the granular layer and orthokeratosis. The epidermal hyperplastic changes resolve later. There may be residual mild superficial dermal fibrosis with persistence of papillary dermal capillary dilatation

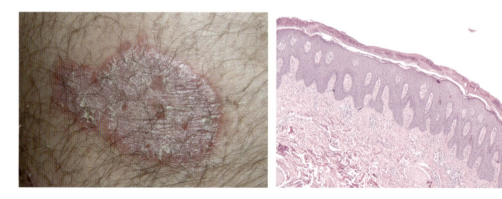

FIGURE 13.3 Plaque psoriasis: clinical and histological features of the late steady-state phase.

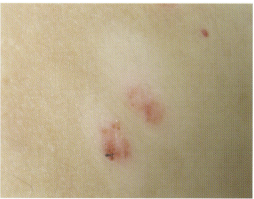 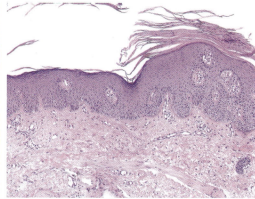

FIGURE 13.4 Plaque psoriasis: clinical and histological features of the phase of resolution.

and tortuosity as the only histopathologic clues to the disease. The clinical resolution of lesions is associated with the return of the abnormal plaque microvessels towards normal.[5]

The microvasculature is of pathologic relevance to psoriasis, and excessive dermal angiogenesis is a characteristic feature.[6] Until now, it is still a matter of debate if the early changes in psoriasis are referred to the epidermis or to the vascular supply. There is evidence that epidermal hyperplasia cannot occur without vascular proliferation, represented by an abnormal growth of endothelial cells in the microvessels around the perilesional skin.[7] The starting event of psoriasis seems to be the initial vasodilatation that is accompanied by exudates of inflammatory cells and serum in the papilla.[8] Nevertheless, some authors have provided evidence that keratinocyte-derived pro-angiogenic cytokines such as interleukin-1 (IL-1) and vascular endothelial growth factor (VEGF) are increased in psoriatic epidermis.[9–10] Furthermore, the fact that epidermal changes may initiate lesions is substantiated by the observation that even nonlesional psoriatic skin shows an enhanced production of cytokines, and appears to be primed for leukocyte adherence.[11]

There is considerable support about the role of tumor necrosis factor-alpha (TNF-α) in expansion of the dermal microvasculature in psoriasis.[4,6,9,12–14] TNF-α is recognized in raising the expression of adhesion molecules and vascular cell adhesion molecules on keratinocytes[14] and in inducing VEGF production, which stimulates endothelial mitogenic activity in the skin.[9] The exhibition of adhesion molecules and chemokines results in the enrollment of additional inflammatory cells to the plaque. The recruited cells can then produce further TNF-α and γ-interferon, potentially amplifying local inflammation and keratinocyte proliferation.[14]

DERMATOSCOPY/ VIDEODERMATOSCOPY FEATURES

A comprehensive evaluation of the cutaneous microvascular structure is possible using different tools, including videocapillaroscopy (VCP) and/or videodermatoscopy (VD) at magnifications usually ranging between ×50 and ×500. A drop of cedar oil is generally used to improve capillary visibility. The glass plate of the videodermatoscope is placed carefully upon the skin to reach a minimal compression of capillaries, which are then easily visualized.

An appropriate knowledge of the normal skin vascular pattern is a prerequisite for recognizing the psoriasis microvessels, which appear different in shape and morphology. The cutaneous microcirculation is organized in two horizontal networks: one is situated 1.5 mm below the skin surface and the other at the dermal-subcutaneous boundary. They are connected by ascending arterioles and descending venules. From the upper layer, arterial capillaries rise to form the dermal capillary loops that represent the nutritive component of the skin circulation.[15] In normal skin, at ×100–×200 VD observation, capillary loops appear with the major axis running perpendicular to the skin surface, and are therefore

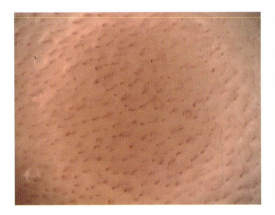

FIGURE 13.5 VD of normal skin: "comma-like" appearance of the capillary loops (×100).

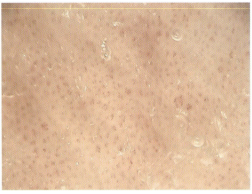

FIGURE 13.6 VD of psoriatic skin: presence of bushy capillaries (×50).

characterized by a "comma-like" appearance inside the dermal papilla (Figure 13.5). The normal capillaroscopic picture differs according to the body areas: in some districts, such as the dorsum of the hand, not all of the capillaries run perpendicular to the skin surface and visibility is not limited to the apical portion; in the forehead, for example, all capillaries run parallel to the skin surface, with a "network" appearance. The evidence of the deep venular sub-papillary plexus depends on the skin transparency.

In psoriasis, the overall organization of the dermal microcirculation is the same as in normal skin. However, it displays many anatomical and physiological changes, mainly described in the intrapapillary portion of the loops. Each papilla continues to be served by a single capillary, but the limbs are twisted along their major axis. The outside endothelial diameters of the loops are also wider (6–17 μm) than the corresponding segments in normal skin (3.5–6 μm). The papillary microvessel changes are homogeneously distributed throughout clinical lesions.[5]

The capillaroscopic picture of plaque psoriasis has been extensively described in the literature,[13,16–18] highlighting the presence in untreated psoriatic skin of many uniformly arranged tortuous and dilated capillaries, appearing as "bushy," with a highly distinctive pattern (Figures 13.6–13.8). Moreover, VD provides additional information about distribution, morphology, and density of capillaries in the psoriatic plaques. In the perilesional skin, capillary loops show a parallel course, with respect to the skin surface, with a lengthened tip directed toward the lesion edges[13] (Figure 13.9). A minimal shift of the probe from the perilesional to normal-appearing skin allows

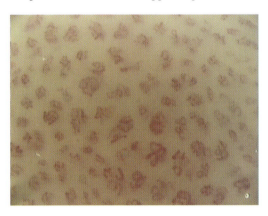

FIGURE 13.7 VD of psoriatic skin: uniformly arranged tortuous and dilated bushy capillaries (×200).

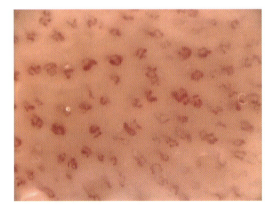

FIGURE 13.8 VD of psoriatic skin: uniformly arranged bushy capillaries (×200).

Inflammatory Diseases

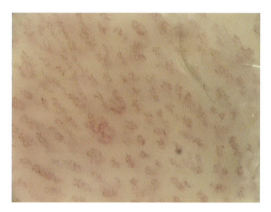

FIGURE 13.9 VD of psoriatic perilesional skin: capillary loops show a parallel course, with respect to the skin surface, with a lengthened tip directed toward the lesion edge (×200).

the visualization of capillary loops that gradually become perpendicular. These studies lead to the recognition of a critical pathogenetic role of angiogenesis in sustaining and spreading out of the psoriasis lesions.

In a study on 105 adult patients affected by clinically or histologically confirmed plaque psoriasis, a total of 177 psoriatic plaques were analyzed and, in all cases, the presence of monomorphic, homogeneously distributed, bushy capillaries, with a mean diameter of 83.9 μm (range 50–146 μm) was observed.[19] For cohort comparison, 50 subjects with atopic dermatitis and 50 with allergic or irritant contact dermatitis were selected and matched with the psoriasis cohort by sex and age. In these patients, the vascular pattern was not specific, showing normal-looking capillaries (25% of cases), slightly dilated capillaries (30% of cases), and/or isolated bushy capillaries (45% of cases).[19]

VD has demonstrated its diagnostic value in clinically doubtful erythematous-desquamative lesions also in pediatric age. In an open comparative study of 24 children with clinical diagnosis of psoriasis, the presence of dilated capillaries with a bushy aspect was seen in all considered plaques, while in children with other erythematous-desquamative disorders VD findings were not specific.[20]

Some studies in small series have considered the use of handheld dermatoscopy (×10 magnification) in psoriasis.[21–23] In the largest study including 300 lesions from 255 patients with solitary red scaly patches or plaques, the main features identified in psoriasis were a homogeneous vascular pattern, red dots, and a light red background, yielding a diagnostic probability of 99% if all three features were present.[23] Red dots were seen in all cases of psoriasis studied. The presence of arborizing vessels was the most valuable negative feature in differentiating psoriasis from basal cell carcinoma.[23]

VD represents a valid noninvasive aid in the diagnosis of psoriasis, particularly in those cases in which the clinical presentation is doubtful. This has been demonstrated in hand, scalp, genital, and inverse psoriasis, in which cases the clinical diagnosis may sometimes be troublesome.

In normal palmo-plantar skin surface VD examination shows at ×100–×200 magnification the presence of capillary loops linearly arranged along the furrows of dermatoglyphics (Figure 13.10). In palmo-plantar psoriasis, these

 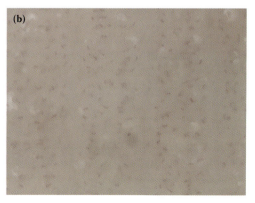

FIGURE 13.10 VD of normal palmar skin surface: presence of capillary loops arranged linearly along the furrows of dermatoglyphics at ×100 (a) and ×200 (b) magnification.

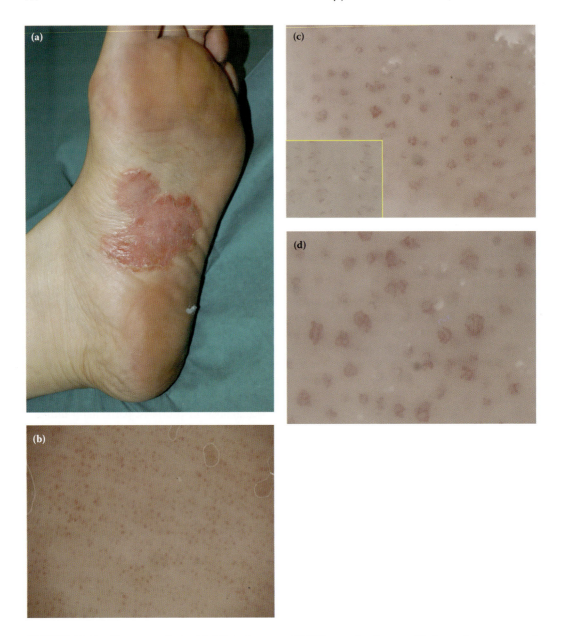

FIGURE 13.11 Plantar psoriasis. (a) Clinical aspect. (b) VD examination at ×50 shows the presence of pinpoint-like capillaries arranged linearly along the furrows of dermatoglyphics. (c) At ×200 the same capillaries appear dilated and tortuous, with a bushy aspect. Insert: normal capillaries at the same magnification. (d) Bushy capillaries at higher magnification (×400).

capillaries appear homogeneously dilated and tortuous, with a bushy aspect[24] (Figure 13.11). A major limitation in this anatomical site, which may interfere with a reliable VD evaluation, is represented by the frequent presence of excessive hyperkeratosis, which may hamper vascular structure analysis; in such cases, VD examination might be performed in residual erythematous areas or after application for 3–4 days of keratolytic creams, such as 30%–50% urea. The

Inflammatory Diseases

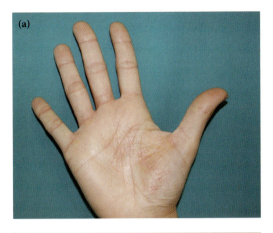

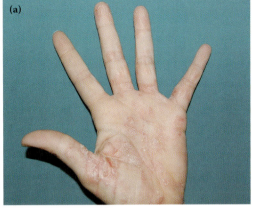

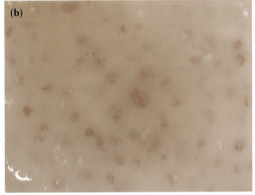

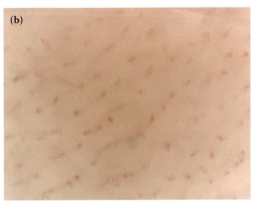

FIGURE 13.12 (a) Palmar dermatosis with no specific clinical features. (b) VD showing the presence of bushy capillaries (×200), suggesting a diagnosis of psoriasis, confirmed by histopathology.

FIGURE 13.13 (a) Palmar dermatosis with no specific clinical features. (b) VD showing no evidence of bushy capillaries (×200). In this case, a diagnosis of psoriasis may be excluded.

efficacy of VD in recognizing palmo-plantar psoriasis has been demonstrated in a series of 32 patients affected by clinically nonspecific, active, and untreated palmar and/or plantar, erythematous, scaly lesions with no other skin involvement.[24] VD was able to identify 15 cases of palmo-plantar psoriasis, as later confirmed by histopathologic examination, showing in all examined fields at ×200 the typical bushy capillaries (Figure 13.12). In the other 17 cases no bushy capillaries were observed and the diagnosis of psoriasis was excluded (Figure 13.13). In these cases, histology showed a pattern consistent with a diagnosis of spongiotic dermatitis.

Psoriatic balanitis is clinically characterized by erythematous nonscaling plaques most commonly located on the glans and under the prepuce.[25] In general, genital psoriasis is part of a more generalized cutaneous disorder, but, in the case of exclusive penile involvement, the correct diagnosis may be troublesome, and several investigations, including skin biopsy, are often necessary. VD examination of glans in healthy subjects shows at ×100 magnification the presence of normal capillary loops (Figure 13.14). Similarly to cutaneous lesions of psoriasis, VD evaluation of psoriasis of the glans shows dilated and tortuous capillaries homogeneously appearing as bushy (Figure 13.15). In this site, because of the absence of scales, the visualization of vascular structures is easy. In a study of 12 patients with balanitis,[26] the typical bushy aspect was observed (×100–×200) only in the 6 patients with biopsy-proven psoriatic

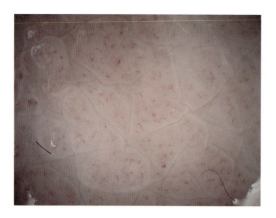

FIGURE 13.14 VD examination of normal glans penis: presence of normal capillary loops (×100).

balanitis (Figure 13.16), while in the remaining cases of nonpsoriatic balanitis (lichen sclerosus, Zoon balanitis, and candidiasis) a nonspecific vascular pattern, consisting of dilated, linear, irregularly distributed capillaries, was evident (Figure 13.17).

Scalp psoriasis and seborrheic dermatitis may be difficult to differentiate. Distinction between the two diseases is obviously relevant for the long-term prognosis, but it may be particularly important in patients with arthritis symptoms. In fact, the presence of skin psoriasis is an important criterion for the diagnosis of psoriatic arthritis, and deciding whether erythematous scaly plaques on the scalp are psoriasis or seborrheic dermatitis may change the interpretation of the rheumatic symptoms. A study of 90 subjects compared capillary morphology in psoriasis, seborrheic dermatitis, and normal skin of the scalp.[27] Scalp psoriasis presented a homogeneous pattern with tortuous and dilated capillaries (appearing as bushes or clews) and a completely disarranged microscopic vascular pattern (Figure 13.18). The capillary loops

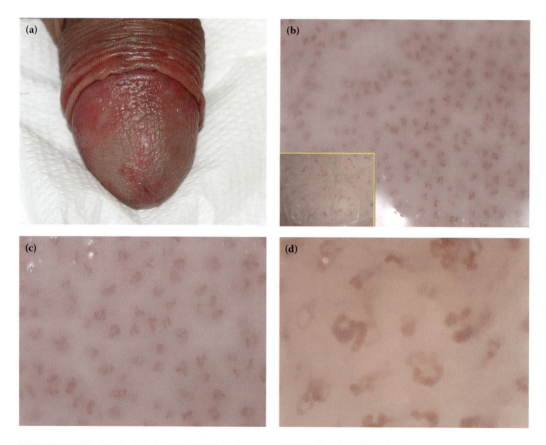

FIGURE 13.15 Psoriatic balanitis. (a) Clinical aspect. (b) VD showing dilated and tortuous capillaries, with a bushy aspect (×100). Insert: normal capillaries at the same magnification. (c) The same bushy capillaries at ×200. (d) Bushy capillaries at higher magnification (×400).

Inflammatory Diseases

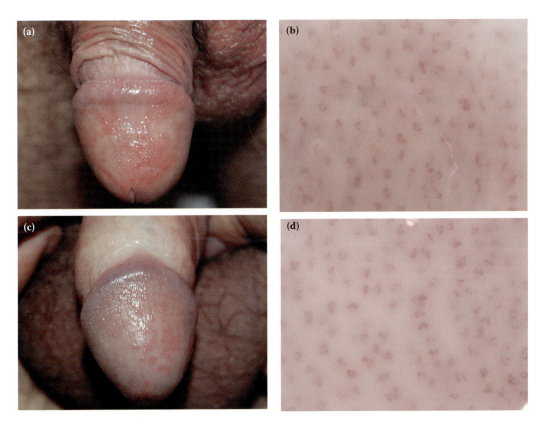

FIGURE 13.16 Psoriatic balanitis. (a–c) Clinical aspect. (b–d) VD showing dilated and tortuous capillaries, with a bushy aspect (×200).

have identical bushy morphology in all scalp locations (Figure 13.19). In contrast, scalp seborrheic dermatitis presented a multiform pattern, with mildly tortuous capillaries and only isolated bushy and mildly dilated capillaries (Figures 13.20-13.21), and with a conserved local microangioarchitecture similar to healthy scalp skin (Figure 13.22). The diameter of capillary bush of scalp psoriasis was much greater than in scalp affected by seborrheic dermatitis or normal scalp skin of healthy subjects. In seborrheic dermatitis, the mean diameter of capillary bush was similar to that of the scalp

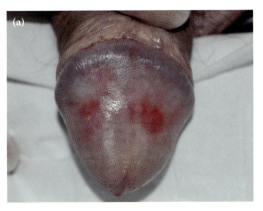
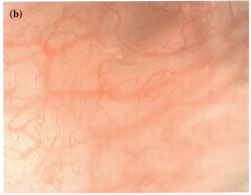

FIGURE 13.17 Zoon balanitis. (a) Clinical aspect. (b) VD showing a nonspecific vascular pattern with a yellowish background color and dilated, linear, irregularly distributed capillaries (×200).

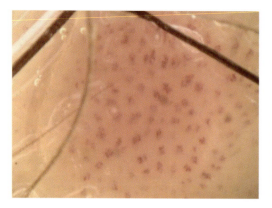

FIGURE 13.18 VD of scalp psoriasis: homogeneous psoriatic pattern with tortuous and dilated capillaries (appearing as bushes or clews) (×100).

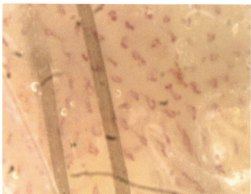

FIGURE 13.21 VD of seborrheic dermatitis: mildly tortuous capillaries and only isolated bushes (×200).

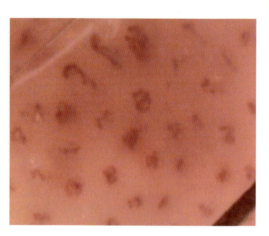

FIGURE 13.19 VD of scalp psoriasis: capillary loops with bushy morphology (×200).

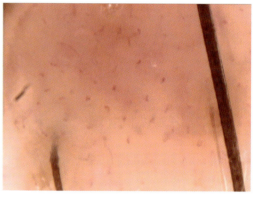

FIGURE 13.22 VD of normal scalp skin of healthy subject (×100).

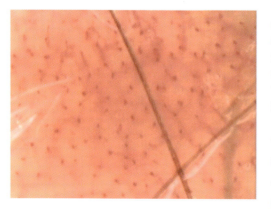

FIGURE 13.20 VD of scalp seborrheic dermatitis: conserved local microscopic vascular pattern similar to healthy scalp skin (×100).

of healthy subjects. Capillary loop density was similar in all conditions.

Finally, VD may also assist in the diagnosis of inverse psoriasis, as demonstrated in a study on 20 patients with erythematous lesions localized to cutaneous body folds, in which the typical bushy pattern was found only in the subjects with clinically and/or histologically confirmed psoriasis.[28]

THERAPEUTIC MONITORING OF PSORIASIS

The role of VD and VCP in psoriasis for *in vivo* therapeutic monitoring is of growing interest, with a number of studies reporting morphological modifications and loop changes after topical and systemic treatments.[16,22,29–33]

In a study, by means of a VD at ×200 magnification, the grossly dilated and tortuous aspect of the untreated psoriatic capillaries appeared to be reduced in 5 patients after the application of tacalcitol ointment 4 µg/g, with a marked simplification of the coiling of the capillary ball occurring after 3 weeks in 2 cases.[16]

With regard to systemic agents, a 3-month treatment period with cyclosporine (4 mg/kg/day) produced a statistical reduction in microcirculatory alterations, assessed by digital capillaroscopy (×300), in 70% of 12 treated subjects, with an average reduction by 64.8% in the "basket" diameter.[29] Modification of the capillaroscopic aspects took place in a progressive manner in all patients, but none returned to a normal capillaroscopic pattern. In another study, 20 patients with moderate-to-severe psoriasis were divided into two groups (A and B) based on PASI score. Group A (PASI >16) was treated with 5 mg/kg/day for 4 weeks and another 4 weeks with 3 mg/kg/day. Group B (PASI 10–16) received 3 mg/kg/day for 8 weeks. At the end of the study, the normalization rate of the vascular pattern, assessed by VD at ×150, was low in both groups (46% and 22%, respectively), despite complete normalization by clinical and ultrasound assessment observed in most cases.[32] Similar results were obtained on patients with moderate-to-severe psoriasis treated with biologicals.[33] In another study, a single infusion of infliximab induced significant changes in morphology of the capillary loops in psoriatic lesions, which appeared less tortuous and dilated, showing an evident reduction in shape and size[31] (Figure 13.23). The number of bushy loops was manifestly reduced, suggesting that infliximab may in part achieve its results by targeting the angiogenetic properties of TNF-α.

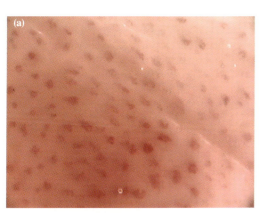

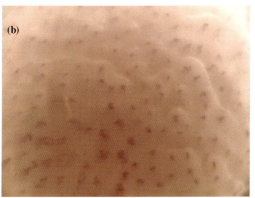

FIGURE 13.23 VD of psoriatic skin at baseline (a) and after a single infusion of infliximab (b): the number of bushy loops is clearly reduced (×200).

REFERENCES

1. Gudjonsson JE, Elder JT. Psoriasis: epidemiology. *Clin Dermatol.* 2007;25(6):535–46.
2. Naldi L, Gambini D. The clinical spectrum of psoriasis. *Clin Dermatol.* 2007;25(6):510–18.
3. Murphy M, Kerr P, Grant-Kels JM. The histopathologic spectrum of psoriasis. *Clin Dermatol.* 2007;25(6):524–28.
4. Creamer D, Allen MH, Sousa A, et al. Localization of endothelial proliferation and microvascular expansion in active plaque psoriasis. *Br J Dermatol.* 1997;136(6):859–65.
5. Hern S, Mortimer PS. In vivo quantification of microvessels in clinically uninvolved psoriatic skin and in normal skin. *Br J Dermatol.* 2007;156(6):1224–29.
6. Micali G, Lacarrubba F, Musumeci ML, et al. Cutaneous vascular patterns in psoriasis. *Int J Dermatol.* 2010;49:249–56.
7. Folkmann J. Angiogenesis in cancer, vascular, rheumatoid and other diseases. *Nat Med.* 1995;1:27–31.
8. Creamer JD, Barker JNWN. Vascular proliferation and angiogenic factors in psoriasis. *Clin Exp Dermatol.* 1995;20:6–9.
9. Detmar M, Brown LF, Claffey KP, et al. Overexpression of vascular permeability factor/vascular endothelial growth factor and its receptors in psoriasis. *J Exp Med.* 1994;180:1141–46.
10. Debets R, Hegmans JPJJ, Troost RJJ, et al. Enhanced production of biologically active interleukin-1α and interleukin-1β by psoriatic epidermal cells ex vivo: Evidence of increased

cytosolic interleukin-1β levels and facilitated interleukin-1 release. *Eur J Immunol.* 1995;25:1624–30.
11. Prens EP, Debets R. Reply to the letter of Li et al. *J Am Acad Dermatol.* 1996;1020–21.
12. Ettehadi P, Greaves W, Wallach D, et al. Elevated tumor necrosis factor-alpha (TNF-α) biological activity in psoriatic skin lesions. *Clin Exp Immunol.* 1994;96:146–51.
13. De Angelis R, Bugatti L, Del Medico P, et al. Videocapillaroscopic findings in the microcirculation of the psoriatic plaque. *Dermatology.* 2002;204:236–39.
14. Krueger JG. The immunologic basis for the treatment of psoriasis with new biologic agents. *J Am Acad Dermatol.* 2002;46:1–23.
15. Braverman IM. The cutaneous microcirculation. *J Invest Derm Symp Proc.* 2000;5:3–9.
16. Strumia R, Altieri E, Romani I, et al. Tacalcitol in psoriasis: A video-microscopy study. *Acta Derm Venereol (Stock).* 1994;Suppl 186;85–87.
17. Fuga GC, Marmo W, Acierno F, et al. Cutaneous microcirculation in psoriasis. A videocapillaroscopic morphofunctional study. *Acta Derm Venereol (Stock).* 1994;186;138.
18. Okada N, Nakatani S, Ozawa K, et al. Video macroscopic study of psoriasis. *J Am Acad Dermatol.* 1991;25:1077–78.
19. Lacarrubba F, Musumeci ML, Ferraro S, et al. A three-cohort comparison with videodermatoscopic evidence of the distinct homogeneous bushy capillary microvascular pattern in psoriasis vs. atopic dermatitis and contact dermatitis. *J Eur Acad Dermatol Venereol.* 2015 Feb 16. doi: 10.1111/jdv.12998.
20. Musumeci ML, Lacarrubba F, Verzì AE, Micali G. Evaluation of the vascular pattern in psoriatic plaques in children using videodermatoscopy: An open comparative study. *Pediatr Dermatol.* 2014;31(5):570–74.
21. Vázquez-López F, Manjon-Haces JA, Maldonado-Seral C, et al. Dermoscopic features of plaque psoriasis and lichen planus: New observation. *Dermatology.* 2003;207:151–56.
22. Vázquez-López F, Marghoob AA. Dermoscopic assessment of long-term topical therapies with potent steroids in chronic psoriasis. *J Am Acad Dermatol.* 2004;51:811–13.
23. Pan Y, Chamberlain AJ, Bailey M, et al. Dermatoscopy aids in the diagnosis of the solitary red scaly patch or plaque-features distinguishing superficial basal cell carcinoma, intraepidermal carcinoma and psoriasis. *J Am Acad Dermatol.* 2008;59:268–74.
24. Micali G, Nardone B, Scuderi A, Lacarrubba F. Videodermatoscopy enhances the diagnostic capability of palmar and/or plantar psoriasis. *Am J Clin Dermatol.* 2008;9:119–22.
25. Buechner SA. Common skin disorders of the penis. *BJU Int.* 2002;9:498-506.
26. Lacarrubba F, Nasca MR, Micali G. Videodermatoscopy enhances diagnostic capability in psoriatic balanitis. *J Am Acad Dermatol.* 2009;61:1084–86.
27. Rosina P, Zamperetti MR, Giovannini A, Girolomoni G. Videocapillaroscopy in the differential diagnosis between psoriasis and seborrheic dermatitis of the scalp. *Dermatology.* 2007;214:21–24.
28. Musumeci ML, Lacarrubba F, Catalfo P, et al. Videodermatoscopy evaluation of the distinct vascular pattern of psoriasis also improves diagnostic capability for inverse psoriasis: a paired-comparison study. *G Ital Dermatol Venereol.* 2015 Sep 17.
29. Stinco G, Lautieri S, Valente F, Patrone P. Cutaneous vascular alterations in psoriatic patients treated with cyclosporine. *Acta Derm Venereol.* 2007;87:152–54.
30. Iorizzo M, Dahadah M, Vincenzi C, Tosti A. Videodermoscopy of the hyponychium in nail bed psoriasis. *J Am Acad Dermatol.* 2008;58:714–15.
31. De Angelis R, Gasparini S, Bugatti L, Filosa G. Early videocapillaroscopic changes of the psoriatic skin after anti-tumour necrosis factor-alpha treatment. *Dermatology.* 2005;210:241–43.
32. Musumeci ML, Lacarrubba F, Fusto CM, Micali G. Combined clinical, capillaroscopic and ultrasound evaluation during treatment of plaque psoriasis with oral cyclosporine. *Int J Immunopathol Pharmacol.* 2013;26:1027–33.
33. Micali G, Lacarrubba F, Santagati C, et al. Clinical, ultrasound, and videodermatoscopy monitoring of psoriatic patients following biological treatment. *Skin Res Technol.* 2015 Oct 9. doi: 10.1111/srt.12271.

14 Inflammatory diseases
Lichen planus

Francisco Vázquez-López and Felipe Valdes Pineda

DEFINITION

Lichen planus (LP), or lichen ruber planus, is an idiopathic inflammatory disease that involves the skin, hair, nails, and mucous membranes.

EPIDEMIOLOGY/ETIOPATHOGENESIS

Although its incidence varies depending on geographic area, cutaneous LP has been reported to affect from about 1% of the general population with two-thirds of patients developing the disease between the ages of 30 and 60 years. Mucosal involvement, particularly oral lesions, may be observed in up to 75% of patients. The etiology of LP is not entirely understood. It is thought to be an immunologically T-cell-mediated disorder resulting in damage to basal keratinocytes that express altered selfantigens on their surface.

CLINICAL PRESENTATION/DIAGNOSIS

The diagnosis of LP is generally clinical. It is characterized by violaceous papules and plaques. The four Ps (purple, polygonal, pruritic, papule) are used to recall the symptoms and skin features that characterize LP. The surface of the lesions generally shows the pathognomonic Wickham striae (WS) that correspond to white lines or dots seen on the top of the lesions, which recall those observed in the oral mucosa.[1] WS cannot be recognized with the standard visual inspection in all patients, although it can be rendered more evident by painting the lesions with oil and by examining them with a magnifying lens. Postinflammatory hyperpigmentation (ashy dermatosis, LP pigmentosus, dyscromic and pigmented actinic LP, LP with hyperpigmentation) is typical in late LP lesions; it may be persistent and disturbing for the patients.

Histologically, active papules of LP show a compact orthokeratosis above the zones of wedge-shaped hypergranulosis (centered around acrosyringia and acrotrichia), irregular acanthosis, and damage to the basal cell layer. In addition, a bandlike lympho-hystiocitic dermal infiltrate in close approximation to the epidermis can be demonstrated (Figure 14.1).[2] In pigmented LP, histopathology shows the presence of melanophages in the dermis (Figure 14.2).

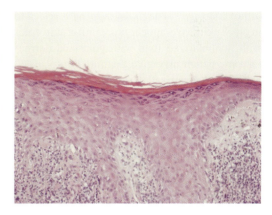

FIGURE 14.1 Typical histopathological picture of lichen planus.

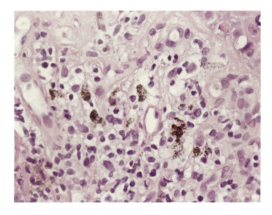

FIGURE 14.2 Pigmented lichen planus: histopathology shows melanophages in the dermis of a long-standing lesion, corresponding to dermatoscopic gray-blue granules.

DERMATOSCOPY/ VIDEODERMATOSCOPY FEATURES

LP discloses specific and pathognomonic dermatoscopic features. It was, in 2001, the first inflammatory skin disease for which dermatoscopy was found to be of value.[3] In conjunction with history and clinical examination, this noninvasive technique is useful for diagnosing and evaluating LP in daily practice in several ways (Table 14.1).

Dermatoscopic analysis of LP lesions requires the knowledge of nonvascular and vascular structures (Table 14.2).

The whitish WS represent the main dermatoscopic feature of LP, a sensitive and specific criterion for the diagnosis.[4–5] WS are visualized as pearly whitish structures (Figures 14.3–14.6) and histopathologically correspond to compact orthokeratosis.[1–2] They may appear blue-white in black skin.[6] WS appear more uniform in color with nonpolarized than with polarized dermatoscopy, which may give them an "unfocused" appearance. Polarized dermatoscopes allows for better recognition of deeper structures (vasculature, dermal pigment, fibrosis) but for worse recognition of the superficial layers of the epidermis.[7]

TABLE 14.1
Clinical value of dermatoscopy in lichen planus lesions

1. **Diagnosis of LP**
   - Enhances recognition of WS
   - Facilitates diagnosis of LP in patients with black skin
   - Facilitates the discrimination of LP from erythematosquamous and granulomatous skin disorders (psoriasis, spongiotic dermatitis, lichenoid sarcoidosis)
   - Facilitates differential diagnosis of genital skin lesions
   - Improves discrimination when coexistence of LP with other diseases
2. **Monitoring of patients with LP**
   - Reveals patterns of pigmentation likely related to prognosis
3. **Clinical teaching**
   - Improves clinical teaching to medical students and residents by linking clinical and histopathological data (sub-elementary lesions)

In addition to the WS, peripheral capillaries (rounded or lineal) and dermal pigment can also be visualized, with variations according to evolution of the lesions (see later discussion).[8–13] Rarely, a rainbow-like pattern, which is considered indicative of Kaposi's sarcoma, may be observed in LP lesions.[14] Dermatoscopic vascular findings in LP have no diagnostic value.

Dermatoscopic findings of cutaneous LP vary according to the lesion's evolution. *Initial LP lesions (round, pink papules)* show small, round WS centered by a yellow-brown dot, which may correspond to vacuolar alterations of basal keratinocytes and to spongiosis in the spinous zone.[2] *Mature LP lesions (violaceous papules or plaques)* (Figures 14.3–14.6) remain isolated or become confluent in reticular networks. WS become polymorphic, showing thin ("comblike" spikes) or broad arboriform projections of the border. Several types of WS can be recognized: round WS, linear WS, arboriform WS, reticular WS, and annular WS. In this phase, the central yellow-brown area disappears and prominent peripheral linear, radial capillaries surround the WS contour, intermingled with the projections of the border. Less characteristic round vessels can also be seen. *Evolved LP lesions* show WS with decreasing, less prominent peripheral vessels. Pigmented structures begin to appear, surrounding the WS contour. Long-standing lesions show pigmented structures, with or without WS devoid of capillaries, according to their duration and the intensity of the inflammatory process.

With regard to clinical variants, *annular LP* appears most commonly in the groin and axillary area, and dermatoscopy of the active border shows WS, capillaries, or pigmented structures according to their duration (Figure 14.7). *Hypertrophic LP* shows at dermatoscopy comedo-like structures filled with yellow plugs or round corneal structures ("corn pearls") in addition to WS and vascular findings (Figure 14.8). In *postinflammatory hyperpigmentation of LP*, ashy or brown macules (Figures 14.9–14.11) show at dermatoscopy homogeneous, structureless, light brown areas devoid of granularity, which seem to correlate with a shorter duration, or granular pigmentation, which corresponds to pigment-laden dermal melanophages and seems to persist longer. Granular pigment consists of fine or coarse, gray-blue or brown, clustered,

Inflammatory Diseases

TABLE 14.2
Dermatoscopic semiology of LP lesions

Dermatoscopic Structures	Morphology	Histopathological Correlation	Significance
Wickham striae	Whitish striae (round, linear, reticular, annular)	Orthokeratosis above wedge-shaped hypergranulosis and acanthosis	Diagnosis of LP (sensitive and specific)
Vessels	Linear	Subpapillary vessels	Diagnosis of LP
	Round	Papillary vessels	(adjunctive features)
Postinflammatory hyperpigmentation	Granular • peripherical • centrally located ("ashy-holes")	Dermal melanophages	Related to a longer duration of the hyperpigmentation
	Homogeneous		Related to a shorter duration of the hyperpigmentation
Comedo-like "corn" pearls		Follicular plugs	Observed in hypertrophic LP lesions

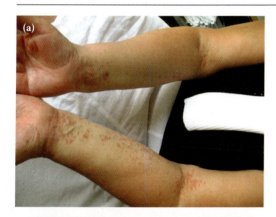

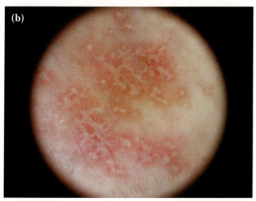

FIGURE 14.3 Lichen planus. (a) Active, well developed, violaceous papules and plaques located on the arms. (b) Dermatoscopy showing a polygonal network of pathognomonic, Wickham striae surrounded by red capillaries (×10).

round dots or globules, within or not light brown discolorations. They may be located centrally within some rounded WS ("ashy-holes") or outline the WS contour in a striking regular distribution.

Dermatoscopy also may be useful for monitoring the evolution of LP lesions and for the differential diagnosis with other similar conditions. Plaque-psoriasis (PP) and LP are not always well differentiated clinically and may even coexist.[4] WS are always absent in PP, which shows multiple, uniformly sized and distributed round vessels.[4–5,15] At low magnification (×10) they appear as red dots (Figure 14.12); by increasing the degree of magnification (stereomicroscope, videodermatoscope) they are really seen as tortuous loops (described as twisted, coiled, glomerular, hairpin-like, or bushy capillaries). The vessels may have a more oblique course and are less coiled at the periphery than at the center of the plaques (Figure 14.13). The subpapillary horizontal vascular plexus is not seen with any magnification, being hidden by the epidermal hyperplasia, unless atrophy secondary to topical steroid treatment develops.[16] Dermatoscopy enhances the differentiation of LP from skin tumors that clinically mimic it, such as Bowen's disease, characterized by red dots, and superficial basal cell carcinoma,[17–20] typified by linear and micro-arborizing vessels,

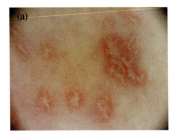 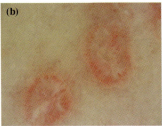 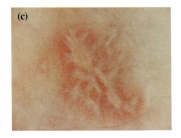

FIGURE 14.4 Dermatoscopy of active lichen planus lesions. (a) Wickham striae contours show broad ramifications, which have a reticular configuration in the largest lesion. They are surrounded by radial capillaries. (b–c) Digitally zoomed images: Wickham striae present projections of the border ("comb-like" appearance), intermingled with defined lineal capillaries (original magnification: ×10).

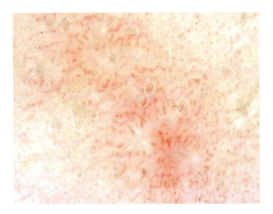

FIGURE 14.5 Dermatoscopy of lichen planus lesions showing radial, linear capillaries. Round vessels can also be present but are less characteristic (×10).

multiple erosions and, in some cases, pigmented structures.[20] Dermatoscopy is also useful for discriminating between LP and lichenoid sarcoidosis, which reveals the structure termed as yellow patches[21–22] (see Chapter 20 for more details). Finally, dermatoscopy improves recognition LP of the genital area, facilitating discrimination from genital warts, balanitis, and psoriasis.[23]

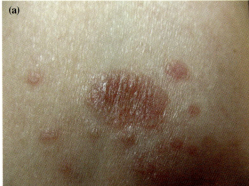

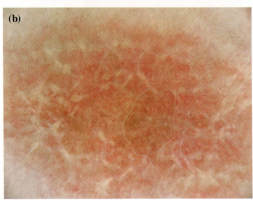

FIGURE 14.6 Active lichen planus plaque. (a) Clinical aspect. (b) Dermatoscopy revealing round and linear Wickham striae configured in a well-developed white, polygonal network, most prominent in the periphery, and outlined by radial capillaries. Some Wickham striae show yellow-brown areas (×10).

Inflammatory Diseases

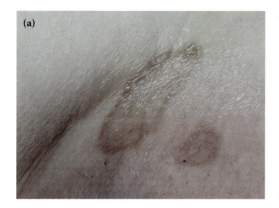

FIGURE 14.7 (a) Long-standing annular lichen planus of the axillary region. (b) Dermatoscopy revealing a granular pigment deposition in the border (digitally zoomed image; original magnification: ×10).

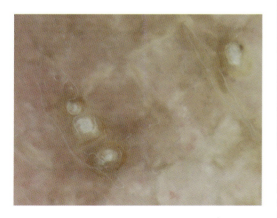

FIGURE 14.8 Dermatoscopy of longstanding, hypertrophic lichen planus plaque showing comedo-like structures filled with yellow plugs or round yellow corneal structures ("corn-pearls") (digitally zoomed image; original magnification: ×10).

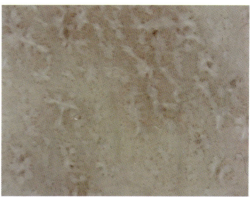

FIGURE 14.9 Dermatoscopy of long-standing, pigmented lichen planus lesion revealing granular pigment outlining the contour of polygonal Wickham striae (×10).

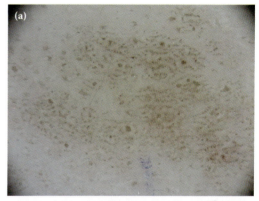

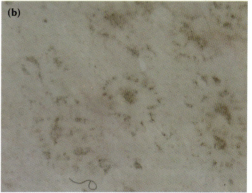

FIGURE 14.10 Dermatoscopy of pigmented lichen planus lesions. Granular pigment consists of fine or coarse, gray-blue or brown round dots or globules that may be centrally or peripherically located according to Wickham striae. Pigment granules appear central within rounded Wickham striae ("ashy-holes") or outlining the Wickham striae contour in a striking regular distribution. (a) ×10. (b) Digitally zoomed image.

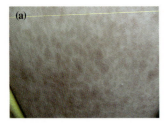  

FIGURE 14.11 Ashy dermatosis related to lichen planus. (a) Clinical aspect. (b) Dermatoscopy showing pigment granules located within homogeneous brown discolorations (×10). (c) Coarse and fine gray-blue and brown globules are better visualized by increasing the magnification with digital zoom.

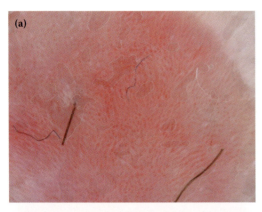

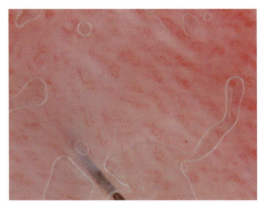

FIGURE 14.13 Dermatoscopy of plaque psoriasis: the capillary loops are less coiled at the periphery of the plaque (digitally zoomed image).

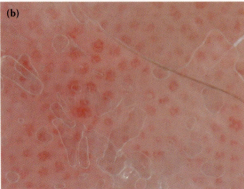

FIGURE 14.12 (a) Dermatoscopy of a psoriatic plaque revealing multiple, uniformly sized and distributed rounded vessels (dots/globules) (×10). (b) A high degree of digital zoom reveals that these apparently rounded vessels are indeed convoluted, "coiled" capillaries.

REFERENCES

1. Rivers JK, Jackson R, Orizaba M. Who was Wickham and what are his striae? *Int J Dermatol.* 1986;25:611–13.
2. Ragaz A, Ackerman AB. Evolution, maturation, and regression of lesions of lichen planus. New observations and correlations of clinical and histologic findings. *Am J Dermatopathol.* 1981;3:5–25.
3. Vázquez-López F, Alvarez-Cuesta C, Hidalgo-García Y, Pérez-Oliva N. The handheld dermatoscope improves the recognition of Wickham striae and capillaries in Lichen planus lesions. *Arch Dermatol.* 2001;137:1376.

4. Vázquez-López F, Manjón-Haces JA, Maldonado-Seral C, et al. Dermoscopic features of plaque psoriasis and lichen planus: New observations. *Dermatology.* 2003;207:151–56.
5. Lallas A, Giacomel J, Argenziano G, et al. Dermoscopy in general dermatology: Practical tips for the clinician. *Br J Dermatol.* 2014;170:514–26.
6. Tan C, Min ZS, Xue Y, Zhu WY. Spectrum of dermoscopic patterns in lichen planus: a case series from China. *J Cutan Med Surg.* 2014;18:28–32.
7. Pan Y, Gareau DS, Scope A, et al. Polarized and nonpolarized dermoscopy: The explanation for the observed differences. *Arch Dermatol.* 2008;144:828–29.
8. Lallas A, Kyrgidis A, Tzellos TG, et al. Accuracy of dermoscopic criteria for the diagnosis of psoriasis, dermatitis, lichen planus and ptyriasis rosea. *Br J Dermatol.* 2012;166:1198–205.
9. Vázquez-López F, Gómez-Díez S, Sánchez J, Pérez-Oliva N. Dermoscopy of active lichen planus. *Arch Dermatol.* 2007;143:1092.
10. Zalaudek I, Argenziano G, Di Stefani A, et al. Dermoscopy in general dermatology. *Dermatology.* 2006; 212:7–18.
11. Vazquez-López F, Marghoob A, Kreusch J. Other uses of dermoscopy. In: *Atlas of Dermoscopy.* Marghoob AA, Braun RP, Kopf AW, Eds. London: Taylor & Francis, 2005: 299–306.
12. Vázquez-López F, Maldonado-Seral C, López-Escobar M, Pérez-Oliva N. Dermoscopy of pigmented lichen planus lesions. *Clin Exp Dermatol.* 2003;28:554–55.
13. Vázquez-López F, Vidal AM, Zalaudek I. Dermoscopic subpatterns of ashy dermatosis related to lichen planus. *Arch Dermatol.* 2010;146:110.
14. Vázquez-López F, García-García B, Rajadhyaksha M, Marghoob AA. Dermoscopic rainbow pattern in non-Kaposi sarcoma lesions. *Br J Dermatol.* 2009;161:474–75.
15. Vázquez-López F, Zaballos P, Fueyo-Casado A, Sánchez-Martín J. Adermoscopy subpattern of plaque-type psoriasis: Red globular rings. *Arch Dermatol.* 2007;143:1612.
16. Vázquez-López F, Marghoob A. Dermoscopic assessment of long-term topical therapies with potent steroids in chronic psoriasis. *J Am Acad Dermatol.* 2004;51:811–13.
17. Pan Y, Chamberlain AJ, Bailey M, et al. Dermatoscopy aids in the diagnosis of the solitary patch or plaque-features distinguishing superficial basal cell carcinoma, intraepidermal carcinoma and psoriasis. *J Am Acad Dermatol.* 2008;59:268–74.
18. Zalaudek I, Argenziano G, Leinweber B, et al. Dermoscopy of Bowen's disease. *Br J Dermatol.* 2004;150:1112–16.
19. Zalaudek I, Giacomel J, Schmid K, et al. Dermatoscopy of facial actinic keratosis, intraepidermal carcinoma, and invasive squamous cell carcinoma: A progression model. *J Am Acad Dermatol.* 2012;66:589–97.
20. Giacomel J, Zalaudek I. Dermoscopy of superficial basal cell carcinoma. *Dermatol Surg.* 2005;31:1710–13.
21. Vazquez-Lopez F, Palacios-Garcia L, Gomez-Diez S, Argenziano G. Dermoscopy for discriminating between lichenoid sarcoidosis and lichen planus. *Arch Dermatol.* 2011; 147:1130.
22. Eirís N, Vázquez-López F, Palacios-García L, et al. Value of dermoscopy for the differential diagnosis of Wolf's post herpetic isotopic response. *Australas J Dermatol.* 2015;56:29–31.
23. Dong H, Shu D, Campbell TM, et al. Dermatoscopy of genital warts. *J Am Acad Dermatol.* 2011;64:859–64.

15 Inflammatory diseases
Common urticaria and urticarial vasculitis

Francisco Vázquez-López and Felipe Valdes Pineda

DEFINITION

Common urticaria (CU) includes a heterogeneous group of disorders characterized by short-lived (few hours) swellings of the skin and mucosa. Urticarial vasculitis (UV) is a variety of urticaria characterized by papular lesions that persist for more than 24 hours.

EPIDEMIOLOGY/ETIOPATHOGENESIS

CU is a common disease, with a prevalence of about 1%–5% in the general population. Although about 50% of cases can be ascribed to allergy, infections, autoimmunity, or other causes, most often CU remains idiopathic. Clinical manifestations are due to a local increase in permeability of capillaries and venules for activation of mast cells containing pro-inflammatory mediators, mainly histamine. UV is a rare disorder. While only approximately 5% of patients with chronic urticaria have UV, this distinction is important because it may be associated with an underlying connective tissue disease. UV is considered to be a type III hypersensitivity immune reaction, with deposition of immune complexes in blood vessels and other tissues.

CLINICAL PRESENTATION/DIAGNOSIS

CU presents acute or chronic (duration of the eruptions >6 weeks) transient wheals histologically characterized by dermal or subcutaneous edema and a sparse or dense perivascular lymphocytic infiltrate, intermingled with neutrophils and eosinophils. In contrast, UV is characterized by urticariform papules or plaques with histopathologic features of leukocytoclastic vasculitis: fibrinoid deposits in the vessels walls, nuclear dust, neutrophilic infiltrates, and slight to moderate extravasation of erythrocytes[1–2] (Figure 15.1). UV presents clinically with urticariform lesions, but each individual papule persists more than 24 hours. Lesions may reveal more or less evident purpuric areas that resolve with residual discoloration. Angioedema may also be present. Systemic symptoms may appear in UV (arthralgia or arthritis, abdominal pain, nephropathy, peripheral neuropathy, asthma, uveitis). A small subset of patients with UV present with hypocomplementemic UV syndrome; they have the propensity to have more severe multi-organ involvement and frequently develop systemic lupus erythematous.[3–4]

Clinical characteristics of UV overlap with those of CU; consequently, UV could be underdiagnosed. The diagnosis of UV is a challenge and requires a skin biopsy. To differentiate between the disorders, nuclear dust and dermal hemorrhage have been considered the most specific differential histopathologic criteria for UV.[1–2]

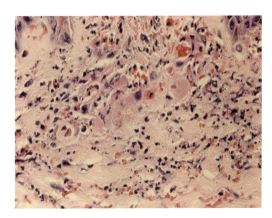

FIGURE 15.1 Urticarial vasculitis lesion presenting histopathologic features of leukocytoclastic vasculitis: fibrinoid deposits in the vessels walls, nuclear dust, neutrophilic infiltrates, and slight to moderate extravasation of erythrocytes.

DERMATOSCOPY/ VIDEODERMATOSCOPY FEATURES

Dermatoscopy, in conjunction with history and clinical examination, is a useful first-line screening tool for discriminating between CU (Figures 15.2–15.5) and UV (Figures 15.6–15.7).[5–11] Dermatoscopic differentiation between the two entities requires the knowledge of both vascular and purpuric structures[5–11] (Table 15.1).

Recognition of *vascular structures* is crucial for evaluating CU (Figures 15.3–15.5). It is important to avoid excessive pressure on the lesion when performing nonpolarized dermatoscopy, as occlusion and lack of visualization of the vessels may occur. Dermal vessels observed at standard magnification (×10) may be seen as round or oval structures. Round structures (vertically oriented papillary

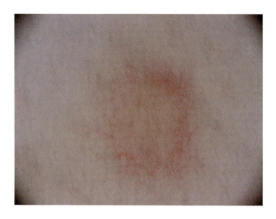

FIGURE 15.4 Dermatoscopy of a common urticaria wheal: peripheral red network of linear vessels surrounding a central negative area in which the vessels are obscured by a prominent edema (×10).

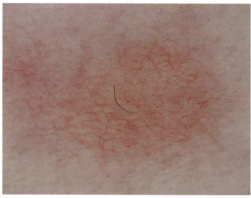

FIGURE 15.5 Dermatoscopy of common urticaria wheal: some ectatic round vessels along the course of the linear vessels are evident. This vascular finding must be differentiated from true purpuric structures (×10).

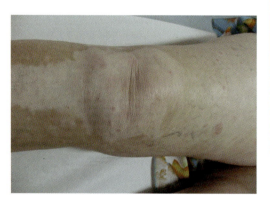

FIGURE 15.2 Common urticaria: transient lesions (wheals) of in a patient with vitiligo.

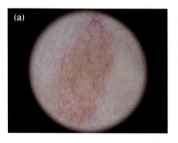
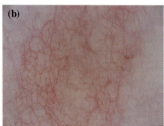
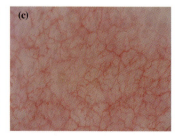

FIGURE 15.3 (a) Polarized dermatoscopy of a common urticaria wheal disclosing a well circumscribed area with a red network of linear vessels (×10). (b–c) Images at greater magnifications, disclosing an irregular network of linear vessels, which corresponds to transiently dilated, horizontally oriented dermal capillaries (digitally zoomed images).

Inflammatory Diseases

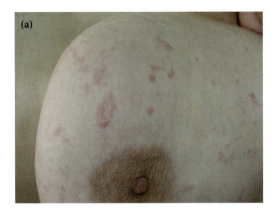

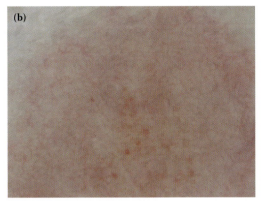

FIGURE 15.6 Urticarial vasculitis. (a) Clinically, the lesions do not show purpuric areas. (b) Polarized dermatoscopy of a papule reveals blurred purpuric globules (×10).

vessels) may be dotted/punctate/pinpointed or globular according to their size (although this differentiation may be difficult to make).

Linear structures (horizontal subpapillary vessels) may be short, long, or arboriform, with a defined or a blurred contour, and may form networks.

Purpuric structures are generally evident in UV (Figures 15.6–15.7). Homogeneous, structureless purpura is observed in non-inflammatory forms of dermal hemorrhage (vessel wall dysfunction or trauma; degeneration of the supporting stroma; bleeding diathesis, coagulation-fibrinolytic disorders, infectious diseases, senile or steroid purpura) (Figure 15.8). Round purpuric dots/globules (PGs) (Figures 15.6, 15.7, 15.9) are derived from perivascular hemorrhage and are associated with different purpuric inflammatory processes (pigmented purpuric dermatoses, arthropods reactions, viral and drug reactions, leucocytoclastic vasculitis, infective organisms); they are blurred and appear within a purpuric background and later within orange-brown patches. Black spots are purpuric/black dots of subcorneal and subungueal purpura and hemorrhagic crusts.

The transient wheals of CU disclose under dermatoscopy a red network of linear vessels without presenting other structures (Figures 15.2–15.5). This standard dermatoscopic pattern corresponds to a process of transient vasodilatation of subpapillary vessels, horizontally oriented. Linear vessels may be associated with dotted vessels (Figure 15.5). In some lesions, red lines may surround structureless areas devoid of vascular findings (Figure 15.4), where the vessels have been

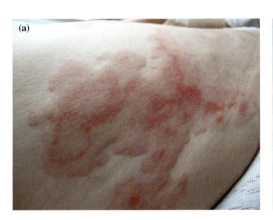 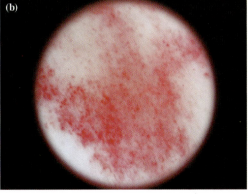

FIGURE 15.7 Urticarial vasculitis. (a) Clinically, lesions consist of raised, urticariform plaques in which the degree of dermal hemorrhage is so severe that some petechiae are evident. (b) Dermatoscopy shows the presence of purpuric globules (×10).

TABLE 15.1
Dermatoscopic semiology of urticaria and urticarial vasculitis

Dermatoscopic Structures		Histopathological Correlation	Significance
Vascular findings	Round vessels Red dots/globules	Papillary vessels	Unspecific (e.g., psoriasis)
	Linear vessels Red short or long lines; arboriform vessels; networks	Subpapillary vessels	Unspecific (e.g., common urticaria)
Purpuric findings	Homogeneous purpuric areas	Dermal hemorrhage	Noninflammatory purpura (e.g., senile purpura)
	Round globular purpuric areas (PG)	Dermal hemorrhage	Inflammatory purpura (e.g., vasculitis) *PG are indicative of UV when confronted with CU*
Black spots			Subcorneal, subungueal purpura

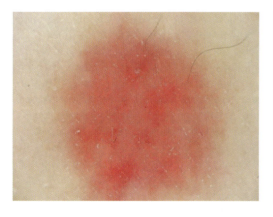

FIGURE 15.8 Dermatoscopy of a noninflammatory form of purpura: homogeneous, structureless purpuric patch devoid of other findings (×10).

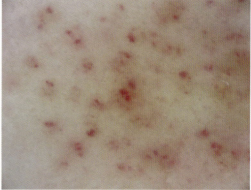

FIGURE 15.9 Dermatoscopy of inflammatory purpura. A lesion of leucocytoclastic vasculitis is shown, disclosing multiple blurred, purpuric globules; some are located within yellow-brown patches (×10).

obscured by a prominent oedema. Purpuric structures are not observed in CU, and red lines disappear after making a pressure on the lesion.

In contrast to CU, persistent urticariform papules of UV characteristically show PGs, which may vary in number according to severity and evolution of the lesions. The degree of dermal hemorrhage in UV lesions is variable. Recognition of PGs allows easy differentiation between UV and CU. Dermatoscopy may be of great value for the screening of lesions with minimal purpuric areas (Figures 15.6); meanwhile, purpura can be clinically evident in some severe cases (Figures 15.7). PGs may or may not appear within purpuric or orange-brown patches. This dermatoscopic pattern corresponds histologically to vasculitis and perivascular extravasation and degradation of red blood cells. In addition, linear vessels may be recognized if hemorrhage is not severe (Figure 15.6).

Red lines and PGs are not specific to CU and UV, respectively, but their recognition helps in discriminating between them. These structures are easily recognizable even by non-expert observers and after minimal training. Dermatoscopic purpuric structures of UV must be differentiated only from round vessels, occasionally present in CU (Figure 15.5). The ectatic vessels of CU disappear after making a pressure on the lesion, while PGs of UV lesions do not blanch.

It is also of interest that the number of PGs in lesions of UV varies according to time and evolution.[11] Suh and colleagues quantified into four grades the number of PGs present in UV lesions (from 0 to more than 40 PGs). These authors demonstrated that PGs are present even in the most early lesions of UV and that they increase in number in late UV lesions. These authors confirmed therefore that dermatoscopy may be of value for discriminating even the early lesions of UV.

To the best of the authors' knowledge, dermatoscopic studies regarding other urticariform syndromes (such as prolonged urticaria with purpura, urticaria-like neutrophilic dermatosis, neutrophilic urticaria with systemic inflammation, or Schnitzler syndrome) are lacking, although they could be of interest.

In conclusion, dermatoscopic discrimination between CU and UV is based on an unspecific feature (PGs), which is rendered specific for UV when confronted with CU.

REFERENCES

1. Ackerman AB. *Histologic diagnosis of inflammatory skin diseases*. Baltimore: Williams and Wilkins, 1997.
2. Peteiro C, Toribio J. Incidence of leukocytoclastic vasculitis in chronic idiopathic urticaria. Study of 100 cases. *Am J Dermatopathol*. 1989;11:528–33.
3. Aydogan K, Karadogan SK, Adim SB, et al. Hypocomplementemic urticarial vasculitis: A rare presentation of systemic lupus erythematosus. *Int J Dermatol*. 2006;45:1057–61.
4. Rivas González AM, Velásquez Franco J, Pinto Peñaranda LF, Márquez JD. Urticaria vasculítica. *Rev Colomb Reumatol*. 2009; 16:154–66.
5. Vázquez-López F, Maldonado Seral C, Soler-Sánchez T, et al. Surface microscopy for discriminating between common urticaria and urticarial vasculitis. *Rheumatology*. 2003;42:1079–82.
6. Vázquez-López F, Kreusch J, Marghoob AA. Dermoscopic semiology: Further insights into vascular features by screening a large spectrum of nontumoral skin lesions. *Br J Dermatol*. 2004;150:226–31.
7. Vazquez-López F, Marghoob A, Kreusch J. Other uses of dermoscopy. In: *Atlas of Dermoscopy*. Marghoob AA, Braun RP, Kopf AW, Eds. London: Taylor & Francis, 2005: 299–306.
8. Vázquez-López F, Fueyo A, Sánchez-Martín, Pérez-Oliva N. Dermoscopy for the screening of common urticaria and urticaria vasculitis. *Arch Dermatol*. 2008;144:568.
9. Lallas A, Giacomel J, Argenziano G, et al. Dermoscopy in general dermatology: practical tips for the clinician. *Br J Dermatol*. 2014;170:514–26.
10. Vázquez-López F, García-García B, Sánchez-Martín J, Argenziano G. Dermoscopic patterns of purpuric lesions. *Arch Dermatol*. 2010;146:938.
11. Suh KS, Kang DY, Lee KH, et al. Evolution of urticarial vasculitis: A clinical, dermoscopic and histopathological study. *J Eur Acad Dermatol Venereol*. 2014.28:674–75.

16 Inflammatory diseases
Connective tissue diseases

Paolo Rosina

DEFINITION

Connective tissue diseases include a variety of autoimmune disorders characterized by chronic inflammation of the connective tissues.

EPIDEMIOLOGY/ETIOPATHOGENESIS

They are relatively common disorders. The pathogenesis is multifactorial, including both genetic and acquired/environmental factors. The damage to connective tissue is a result of complex immunological reactions involving autogenous antigens. The immune activation against self-antigens is demonstrated by the presence of autoantibodies and autoreactive T-cells.

CLINICAL PRESENTATION/DIAGNOSIS

The main connective tissue diseases involving the skin are represented by systemic sclerosis (SSc), dermatomyositis, and lupus erythematosus. The clinical spectrum is heterogeneous, including skin, vascular, joint, muscolar, and systemic manifestations; often the clinical features overlap. Early diagnosis and treatment is paramount in reducing morbidity and mortality. Investigations mainly include routine blood tests, antinuclear antibodies, muscle enzymes, magnetic resonance imaging, electromyography, nailfold capillary microscopy, and muscle biopsy.

DERMATOSCOPY/ VIDEODERMATOSCOPY FEATURES

The evaluation of the skin microvasculature is important in the evaluation of connective tissue diseases. Capillaroscopy is a noninvasive technique able to analyze the microcirculation in all cutaneous sites.[1] It is characterized by relatively low cost, repeatability, high sensitivity, good specificity, and easy interpretation of results. However, despite the increasing interest in capillary microscopy, there is still a surprising discrepancy between its potential applications and its still limited use in daily practice, above all in dermatology. It is used primarily on nailfolds to diagnose and monitor SSc and dermatomyositis and to distinguish primary from secondary Raynaud's phenomenon (RP).

Nailfold capillary microscopy can be performed with various optical instruments such as the videocapillaroscope, videodermatoscope, stereomicroscope, ophthalmoscope, and also handheld dermatoscope.[2-3] The simplest and most direct way to perform an approximate evaluation of skin microcirculation conditions is with the handheld dermatoscope. It is relatively easy to recognize certain features of microvascular involvement in SSc (giant capillaries, microbleeding), although sensitivity is limited by the low level of magnification (×10).

In normal conditions or in primary RP, the nailfold capillaroscopic pattern shows a regular disposition of the capillary loops along the nailbed (Figure 16.1). By contrast, in subjects suffering from secondary RP, one or more alterations in the capillaroscopic findings (architectural disorganization, enlarged loops, giant capillaries, microhemorrhages, reduction of capillary density, angiogenesis, avascular areas) should suggest a connective tissue disease[4] (Figure 16.2). The capillaroscopic pattern should be carefully evaluated because normal or borderline features are wide as reported in a qualitative and quantitative assessment in healthy volunteers; among morphological changes tortuous (43%), ramified (47%), and bushy capillaries (27%) were the most frequently altered

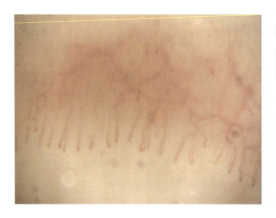

FIGURE 16.1 Nailfold videocapillaroscopy of a healthy subject: regular disposition of the capillary loops along the nailbed (×100).

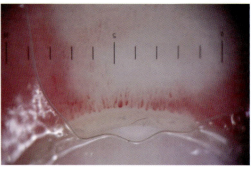

FIGURE 16.3 Nailfold handheld dermatoscopy showing an isolated giant capillary in scleroderma "early" pattern (×20).

capillary types. Megacapillaries and diffuse loss of capillaries were not found in healthy subjects and seem to be of specific diagnostic value for a connective tissue disease.[5]

Patients initially diagnosed with primary RP may shift to secondary during the follow-up. Capillaroscopic analysis twice a year can detect the transition to a secondary form in patients who initially show a normal pattern or nonspecific nailfold capillary abnormalities.

In patients affected by SSc, the most typical nailfold capillary pattern of microangiopathy, the so-called scleroderma pattern (SP), is commonly observed.[6] It is characterized by irregularly enlarged capillaries, giant capillaries (capillary diameter >50 micron of both arteriolar and venular branches), microbleedings, reduced capillary number with avascular areas, capillary architecture disorganization, and ramified capillaries. The giant capillary is pathognomonic of the SP. Three distinct nailfold capillary patterns of microangiopathy have been described in SSc patients: "early," "active," and "late," which do not normally coexist at the same time. "Early" SP is characterized by irregularly enlarged capillaries, a few giant capillaries, and hemorrhages; capillary architecture is almost regular without significant loss of capillaries (Figure 16.3). In the "active" SP pattern, frequent giant capillaries and hemorrhages may be observed with mild loss of capillaries and capillary architecture disorganization (Figures 16.4–16.5). Severe loss of capillaries with a few giant capillaries,

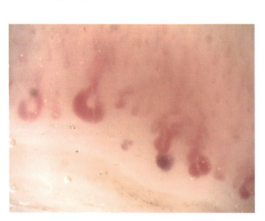

FIGURE 16.2 Nailfold videocapillaroscopy appearance of giant capillary loops in scleroderma (×100).

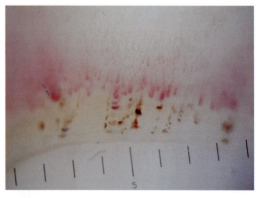

FIGURE 16.4 Nailfold handheld dermatoscopy showing diffuse giant capillaries and hemorrhages in scleroderma "active" pattern (×20).

Inflammatory Diseases

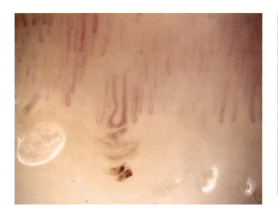

FIGURE 16.5 Nailfold videocapillaroscopy showing giant capillary and hemorrhages in scleroderma "active" pattern (×100).

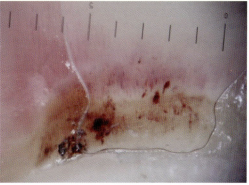

FIGURE 16.7 Nailfold handheld dermatoscopy showing a diffuse hemorrhagic pattern in dermatomiositis (×20).

avascular areas, capillary architecture disorganization, and ramified capillaries are typical abnormalities of "late" SP (Figure 16.6). A nailfold capillaroscopy can help to stage the patient affected by SSc and provides prognostic information. In fact, SPs are related to a disease subset and disease severity affecting different sites than the peripheral circulation, skin, heart, and lungs. SSc patients with "late" capillary pattern show an increased risk for active disease and moderate/severe skin or visceral involvement, compared with patients with early and active patterns.

The capillary features observed in dermatomyositis (Figure 16.7) and in undifferentiated connective tissue disease are generally reported as being of the "scleroderma-like pattern."

In cutaneous discoid lupus erythematosus, tortuous and irregular "bushy" capillaries are already visible with a handheld dermatoscope (Figure 16.8), but in advanced lesions a completely disarranged microangioarchitecture with loss of capillaries (avascular areas) and marked angiogenesis are better observed with capillaroscopy. In subacute lupus erythematosus, polygon irregularities and vessel tortuosity are observed (Figure 16.9). This vascular pattern can be used in differential diagnosis when cutaneous manifestations of lupus erythematosus clinically resemble psoriasis, the last presenting a typical, homogeneous "bushy" pattern (Figure 16.10).

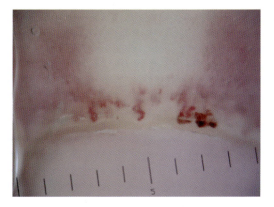

FIGURE 16.6 Nailfold handheld dermatoscopy showing irregular capillaries distribution with a few giant capillaries and avascular area in scleroderma "late" pattern (×20).

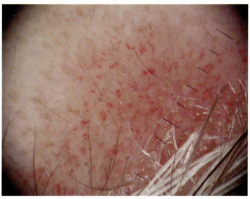

FIGURE 16.8 Handheld dermatoscopy of a plaque of discoid lupus erythematosus showing tortuous and irregular bushy capillaries (×20).

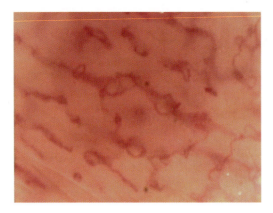

FIGURE 16.9 Videocapillaroscopy of a lesion of subacute lupus erythematosus showing vessel tortuosity (×200).

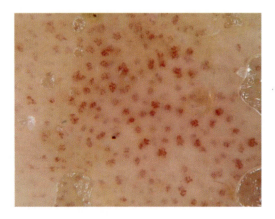

FIGURE 16.10 Videocapillaroscopy of a psoriatic plaque showing homogeneously distributed "bushy" vessel (×100).

REFERENCES

1. Cutolo M, Pizzorni C, Sulli A. Capillaroscopy. *Best Pract Res Clin Rheumatol.* 2005;19:437–52.
2. Bergman R, Sharony L, Schapira D, et al. The handheld dermatoscope as a nail-fold capillaroscopic instrument. *Arch Dermatol.* 2003;139:1027–30.
3. Sontheimer RD. A portable digital microphotography unit for rapid documentation of periungual nailfold capillary changes in autoimmune connective tissue diseases. *J Rheumatol.* 2004;31:539–44.
4. Cutolo M, Grassi W, Matucci Cerinic M. Raynaud's phenomenon and the role of capillaroscopy. *Arthritis Rheum.* 2003;48:3023–30.
5. Hoert C, Kundi M, Katzenschlager R, Hirschl M. Qualitative and quantitative assessment of nailfold capillaries by capillaroscopy in healthy volunteers. *Vasa.* 2012;41:19–26.
6. Caramaschi P, Canestrini S, Martinelli N, et al. Scleroderma patients nailfold videocapillaroscopic patterns are associated with disease subset and disease severity. *Rheumatology.* 2007;46:1566–69.

17 Inflammatory diseases
Rosacea

Paolo Rosina

DEFINITION

Rosacea is a chronic inflammatory skin disorder characterized by erythema, telangiectasias, papules, and pustules, primarily affecting the convexities of the centrofacial area.

EPIDEMIOLOGY/ETIOPATHOGENESIS

It is common, affecting 10%–20% of the middle-aged population with a higher incidence in fair-skinned persons. Several etiologic factors and pathogenetic mechanisms have been proposed. There is a general agreement that rosacea is primarily a vascular disorder characterized by persistent small vessel dilatation and angiogenesis, increased vascular permeability, and vascular hyperreactivity that results in flushing, telangiectasias, papules-pustules, and phyma. Activation of innate immunity (release of cytokines and antimicrobial molecules such as the peptide cathelicidin), exposure to ultraviolet light, neurogenic inflammation, and microbes (such as Demodex mites) are factors currently thought to be relevant in susceptible individuals.[1]

CLINICAL PRESENTATION/DIAGNOSIS

Rosacea involves primarily the cutaneous microcirculation of the central part of the face. The National Rosacea Society Expert Committee (USA) has proposed a classification and staging defining four subtypes (erythematotelangiectatic, papulopustular, phymatous, and ocular), one variant (granulomatous rosacea), and a grading system based on clinical score.[2] There are currently no objective measures or laboratory tests for assessing and monitoring the severity of rosacea, which rests only on clinical judgment. Some studies on rosacea have considered skin color changes as a surrogate measurement of vessel changes.[3–4] The majority of the trials evaluating erythema and telangiectasias have utilized subjective methods of color measurement and vessel changes. The development of instrumental techniques is obviously important for a more reproducible disease assessment and may allow a more rigorous comparison between studies, especially on drug efficacy.

DERMATOSCOPY/VIDEODERMATOSCOPY FEATURES

Videocapillaroscopy has been considered superior to laser-doppler for the clinical investigation of cutaneous microcirculation in various skin diseases[5] and in cosmetic approaches.[6] It may represent a valid adjunctive method in the early identification and measurement of erythemato-telangiectatic rosacea.

Videocapillaroscopy has been used to evaluate qualitative and quantitative micro-vessels alterations of facial rosacea.[7] Thirty patients with erythemato-telangiectatic rosacea were compared with 30 age- and sex-matched patients with facial seborrheic dermatitis and 30 healthy control subjects using an optical probe at ×100 and ×200 magnifications. Parameters analyzed on the cheek area were the background color, morphological (polygon irregularity, vessel tortuosity, neoangiogenesis) parameters, and quantitative parameters (polygon perimeter, mean diameter of telangiectasias and vessels). A regular polygonal net represents the normal distribution of the cutaneous microcirculation on the cheek, with capillary loops projected at the inner and outer part of the polygons (Figure 17.1a). Patients with rosacea showed a reddish background due to the extended vessel dilatation of the subpapillary plexus (Figure 17.1b). In contrast, healthy subjects and patients with

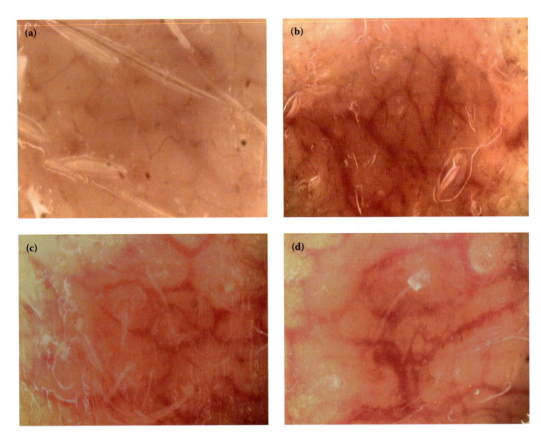

FIGURE 17.1 (a) Videocapillaroscopy of normal facial skin. (b–d) Videocapillaroscopy of rosacea: reddish background, neoangiogenesis, and polygonal net with thickened vessel walls (×100).

seborrheic dermatitis displayed a pink background. Characteristic alterations of skin vessels were observed in facial rosacea, with a pattern distinct from that of facial seborrheic dermatitis. In particular, rosacea showed neoangiogenesis and significantly larger polygons with thickened vessel walls (Figures 17.1c–d), more prominent telangiectasias, and larger mean vessel diameter (Figure 17.2) compared to seborrheic dermatitis. Seborrheic dermatitis displayed more polygon irregularities and vessel tortuosity (Figure 17.3). For all the morphological and quantitative parameters investigated, no substantial differences were noted between male and female patients. In contrast, no alterations were found in the nailfold region, suggesting that rosacea specifically affects the facial microvasculature.

Finally, handheld dermatoscopy has been utilized to evaluate common inflammatory dermatoses of the face:[8] erythemato-telangiectatic rosacea was characterized by a typical pattern of vascular polygons, with prominent linear vessels (Figures 17.4–17.5), as reported in videocapillaroscopy.

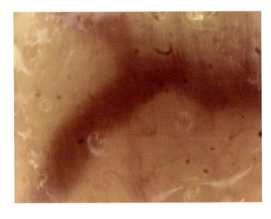

FIGURE 17.2 Videocapillaroscopy of rosacea: telangiectasias (×200).

Inflammatory Diseases

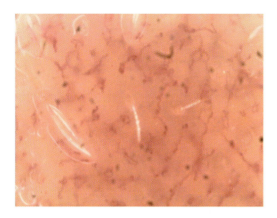

FIGURE 17.3 Videocapillaroscopy of seborrheic dermatitis: marked polygon irregularities and pink background (×100).

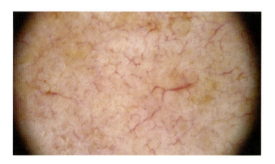

FIGURE 17.4 Handheld dermatoscopy of rosacea: polygonal net (×20).

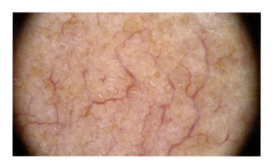

FIGURE 17.5 Handheld dermatoscopy of rosacea: vascular polygons, with prominent linear vessels (×20).

REFERENCES

1. Crawford GH, Pelle MT, James WD. Rosacea: I. Etiology, pathogenesis, and subtype classification. *J Am Acad Dermatol.* 2004;51:327–41.
2. Wilkin J, Dahl M, Detmar M, et al. Standard classification of rosacea: Report of the National Rosacea Society Expert Committee on the classification and staging of rosacea. *J Am Acad Dermatol.* 2004;50:907–12.
3. Bamford JTM, Gessert CE, Renier CM. Measurement of the severity of rosacea. *J Am Acad Dermatol.* 2004;51:697–703.
4. Carpentier PH. New techniques for clinical assessment of the peripheral microcirculation. *Drugs.* 1999;58:17–22.
5. Hern S, Mortimer PS. Visualization of dermal blood vessels—capillaroscopy. *Clin Exp Dermatol.* 1999;24:473–78.
6. Humbert P, Sainthillier JM, Mac-Mary S, et al. Capillaroscopy and videocapillaroscopy assessment of skin microcirculation: dermatologic and cosmetic approaches. *J Cosmet Dermatol.* 2005;4:153–62.
7. Rosina P, Zamperetti MR, Giovannini A, et al. Videocapillaroscopic alterations in erythematotelangiectatic rosacea. *J Am Acad Dermatol.* 2006;54:100–4.
8. Lallas A, Argenziano G, Apalla Z, et al. Dermoscopic patterns of common facial inflammatory skin diseases. *J Eur Acad Dermatol Venereol.* 2014;28:609–14.

18 Inflammatory diseases
Pigmented purpuric dermatoses

Pedro Zaballos Diego

DEFINITION

Pigmented purpuric dermatoses (PPDs), also called purpura simplex or chronic capillaritis, is the generic term for a variety of chronic conditions characterized by petechial and pigmentary macules. They include progressive, pigmented, purpuric dermatosis or Schamberg's disease; pigmented, purpuric lichenoid dermatosis of Gougerot and Blum; eczematoid-like purpura of Doucas and Kapetanakis; purpura annularis telangiectodes or Majocchi's disease; and lichen aureus.[1-3]

EPIDEMIOLOGY/ETIOPATHOGENESIS

PPDs appear more frequently in males, most commonly in the fourth and fifth decades of life. The etiology of PPDs is unknown. Pregnancy and increased venous pressure are important factors in many cases, and triggering factors such as drugs, chemical ingestions, food additives, infections, or underlying hematologic/internal diseases have been described.[1-3]

CLINICAL PRESENTATION/DIAGNOSIS

The various forms of PPD are generally characterized by orange/brown pigmentation (due to hemosiderin deposition likened to cayenne pepper) interspersed with fine-point purpura (due to extravasated red blood cells). They typically occur on the lower limbs (Figures 18.1–18.7) in a symmetrical distribution and often show a benign and self-limited, although chronic, course.

Schamberg's disease (Figures 18.1–18.3) is characterized by usually asymptomatic, chronic, and persistent purpura and petechiae with conspicuous pigmentation located predominantly on the lower limbs. Patients with pigmented, purpuric, lichenoid dermatosis of Gougerot and Blum (Figure 18.4) develop lichenoid papules in addition to purpuric lesions, most often on the legs. Eczematoid-like purpura of Doucas and Kapetanakis (Figure 18.5) or itching purpura has many similarities to Schamberg's disease but is generally more extensive, develops more rapidly, and is characterized by a persistent, intense itch. In Majocchi's disease (Figure 18.6), the lesions tend to be reddish annular macules located on the lower limbs and associated with telangiectasias. Finally, lichen aureus (Figure 18.7) is a localized variant of PPD that is characterized by the appearance of sudden-onset, limited lichenoid papules in association with purpuric lesions, located commonly on the lower limbs, and occasionally on the trunk and the face.

All these disorders may show overlapping clinical and histological features. More unusual PPDs presentations include the itching purpura of Loewenthal as well as linear, granulomatous, quadrantic, transitory, and familial forms.[1-3]

DERMATOSCOPY/VIDEODERMATOSCOPY FEATURES

Under dermatoscopic examination, all forms of PPD show similar findings,[4-6] namely the presence of irregular, round to oval, red dots, globules, and patches, with a red-brownish or red-coppery, diffuse, homogeneous pigmentation in the background (Figures 18.1–18.7). The histopathological correlation of the red-brownish or red-coppery background may be the presence of dermal infiltrate of lymphocytes and histiocytes, extravasated red blood cells, and hemosiderin-laden macrophages. The irregular red dots, globules, and patches, which are not blanched by compression, may correspond to the extravasation of red blood cells and to the

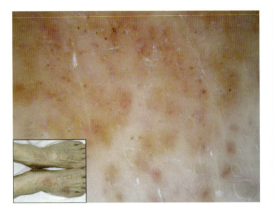

FIGURE 18.1 Dermatoscopy of Schamberg's disease: irregular, round to oval red dots, globules, and patches, with a red-brownish or red-coppery, diffuse, homogeneous pigmentation in the background (×10).

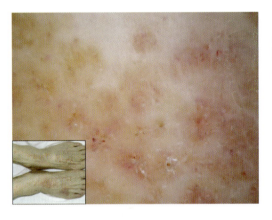

FIGURE 18.2 Dermatoscopy of Schamberg's disease: examination of another area in the same patient shows the presence of vascular structures (×10).

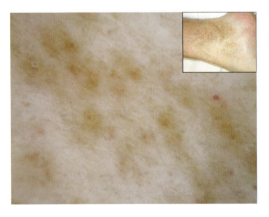

FIGURE 18.3 Dermatoscopy of Schamberg's disease in a more advanced stage: the red-brownish patches predominate (×10).

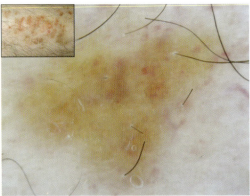

FIGURE 18.4 Dermatoscopy of pigmented purpuric dermatitis of Gougerot and Blum: irregular, round to oval red dots, globules, and patches, with a red-brownish or red-coppery, diffuse, homogeneous pigmentation in the background; a network of brownish to gray interconnected lines can also be observed (×10).

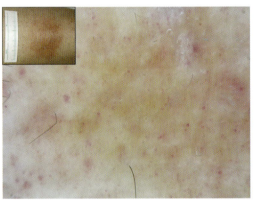

FIGURE 18.5 Dermatoscopy of eczematoid-like purpura of Doucas and Kapetanakis: round to oval red dots and globules and scales, with a red-brownish or red-coppery, diffuse, homogeneous pigmentation in the background (×10).

increased number of blood vessels, some of which are dilated and swollen. In some cases, gray dots and a network of brownish to gray interconnected lines (Figures 18.4 and 18.7) can be observed and correlate, respectively, to hemosiderin-laden macrophages and hyperpigmentation of the basal-cell layer and incontinentia pigmenti in the upper dermis. This pattern of PPDs could be useful to distinguish them from other diseases such as angioma serpiginosum and venous stasis dermatitis. Numerous small, relatively well-demarcated, round to oval red lacunas without the brownish background were

Inflammatory Diseases

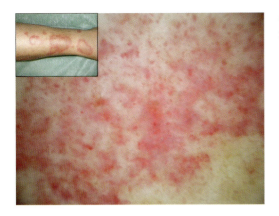

FIGURE 18.6 Dermatoscopy of Majocchi's disease: round to oval red dots, globules and patches, with a scanty, red-brownish, diffuse, homogeneous pigmentation in the background (×10).

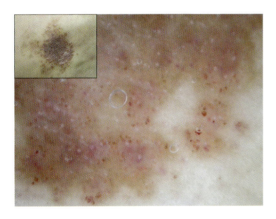

FIGURE 18.7 Dermatoscopy of lichen aureus: irregular, round to oval red dots, globules, and patches, with a red-brownish or red-coppery, diffuse, homogeneous pigmentation in the background; a network of brownish to gray interconnected lines, mainly in the upper part of the lesion, can also be observed (×10).

identified by dermatoscopy in angioma serpiginosum,[7–9] and the presence of glomerular vessels and a scaly surface is the characteristic pattern of venous stasis dermatitis.[10–11]

However, the dermatoscopic pattern observed in PPDs is not pathognomonic, as it can be found in other diseases. Vázquez-López and colleagues found a pattern composed of purpuric or reddish dots and globules in a patchy, orange-brown background in two cases of urticarial vasculitis[12] and also described a similar pattern composed of reddish or brownish globules in diffuse brownish areas in some cases of pigmented lichen planus.[13]

REFERENCES

1. Cox NH, Piette WW. Purpura and microvascular occlusion. In: Burns T, Breathnach S, Cox N, Griffiths C eds. *Rook's Textbook of Dermatology*. Oxford: Blackwell Publishing, 2004. pp. 48.1–48.3.
2. Superficial and deep perivascular inflammatory dermatoses. In: Calonje E, Brenner E, Lazar A, McKee PH. *McKee's Pathology of the Skin with Clinical Correlations*. China: Elsevier Mosby; 2012. pp. 259–280.
3. Sardana K, Sarkar R, Sehgal VN. Pigmented purpuric dermatoses: An overview. *Int J Dermatol*. 2004;43:482–88.
4. Zaballos P, Puig S, Malvehy J. Dermoscopy of pigmented purpuric dermatoses (lichen aureus): A useful tool for clinical diagnosis. *Arch Dermatol*. 2004;140:1290–91.
5. Zalaudek I, Ferrara G, Brongo S, et al. Atypical clinical presentation of pigmented purpuric dermatosis. *J Dtsch Dermatol Ges*. 2006;4:138–40.
6. Zalaudek I, Argenziano G, Di Stefani A, et al. Dermoscopy in general dermatology. *Dermatology*. 2006;212:7–18.
7. Ohnishi T, Nagayama T, Morita T, et al. Angioma serpiginosum: A report of 2 cases identified using epiluminescence microscopy. *Arch Dermatol*. 1999;135:1366–88.
8. Kalisiak MS, Haber RM. Angioma serpiginosum with linear distribution: case report and review of the literatura. *J Cutan Med Surg*. 2008;12:180–83.
9. Ilknur T, Fetil E, Akarsu S, et al. Angioma serpiginosum: dermoscopy for diagnosis, pulsed dye laser for treatment. *J Dermatol*. 2006;33:252–55.
10. Zaballos P, Salsench E, Puig S, Malvehy J. Dermoscopy of venous stasis dermatitis. *Arch Dermatol*. 2006;142:1526.
11. Vázquez-López F, Kreusch J, Marghoob AA. Dermoscopic semiology: Further insights into vascular features by screening a large spectrum of nontumoral skin lesions. *Br J Dermatol*. 2004;150:226–31.
12. Vázquez-López F, Fueyo A, Sánchez-Martín J, Pérez-Oliva N. Dermoscopy for the screening of common urticaria and urticaria vasculitis. *Arch Dermatol*. 2008;144:568.
13. Vázquez-López F, Maldonado-Seral C, López-Escobar M, N Pérez-Oliva. Dermoscopy of pigmented lichen planus lesions. *Clin Exp Dermatol*. 2003;28:554–64.

19 Inflammatory diseases
Pityriasis lichenoides

*Giuseppe Stinco, Francesco Lacarrubba,
Enzo Errichetti, and Giuseppe Micali*

DEFINITION

Pityriasis lichenoides (PL) represents a unique group of uncommon acquired inflammatory skin disorders that include two main variants, pityriasis lichenoides et varioliformis acuta (PLEVA) and pityriasis lichenoides chronica (PLC), and a third much rarer and aggressive form known as febrile ulceronecrotic Mucha-Habermann disease,[1–2] which is not addressed in this chapter.

PLEVA and PLC are actually two ends of the same disease spectrum, and both entities and intermediate variants may coexist. Despite their names, the two conditions mainly differ in their clinical and histological features rather than in the course of the disease, because both disorders last for an average of 18 months.[1,3]

EPIDEMIOLOGY/ETIOPATHOGENESIS

Although PL is more common in children and young adults, it can affect all age, racial, and ethnic groups in all geographic regions with seasonal variation in onset favoring autumn and winter.[1] No significant gender differences exist in the incidence of PL in subjects over 18 years old, while there is a male predominance in the pediatric population.[2] PLC is three to six times more frequent than PLEVA.[3]

Three main etiopathogenetic theories for both PLC and PLEVA have been suggested: inflammatory reactions triggered by infectious agents, inflammatory responses secondary to a T-cell dyscrasia, and immune complex-mediated hypersensitivity vasculitides.[2]

CLINICAL PRESENTATION/DIAGNOSIS

In both PLEVA and PLC, the eruption develops in crops, and consequently appears polymorphic with lesions existing in all stages of development. However, the clinical appearance of the two forms, with particular regard to the morphology of the lesions, is quite different.[1–4]

The initial lesion of PLEVA is a 2- to 3-mm diameter, erythematous macule that quickly evolves into an edematous pink papule, which may centrally become vesiculopustular, hemorrhagic, necrotic, ulcerated, and/or crusted before spontaneously regressing within a matter of weeks (Figure 19.1). Varioliform scars and postinflammatory hyper- and hypopigmentation may result.[1–4] While the lesions are usually asymptomatic, sometimes they may itch and/or burn.[2,4] The most commonly involved sites are trunk, thighs, and upper arms, especially the flexural aspects. The palms and soles are less commonly affected, while the face and scalp are usually spared; mucosal necrotic or erythematous lesions may be present. Rarely, constitutional symptoms such as fever, headache, malaise, and arthralgia may precede or accompany the onset of PLEVA.[1,4]

The typical lesion of PLC is an asymptomatic, small, firm, 3- to 10-mm diameter, erythematous papule that develops a reddish-brown hue and a centrally adherent micaceous scale that may be detached by gentle scraping to reveal a shining pinkish-brown surface (a characteristic diagnostic finding) (Figure 19.2). Over a period of a few weeks, the papule flattens and the scale separates spontaneously to leave a hyper- or hypopigmented macule. PLC usually involves trunk and proximal portions of the extremities,

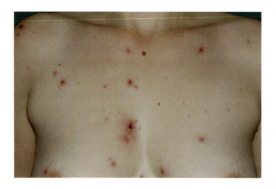

FIGURE 19.1 PLEVA: multiple erythematous papules, some of them covered by necrotic crusts.

but acral and segmental distributions have also been reported.[1–3]

The histopathologic findings of PLEVA and PLC are similar, although in the former the changes are typically more severe.[5] In particular, PLEVA lesions are characterized by a wedge-shaped superficial and deep dermal lymphohistiocytic infiltrate, dermal edema, diffuse disappearance of the dermal-epidermal junction, perivascular and intraepidermal extravasation of erythrocytes, confluent parakeratosis, thinning of the granular layer, ballooning of keratinocytes, intraepidermal vesiculation, and necrosis of keratinocytes. While the endothelial cells are often blurred or swollen, fibrinoid necrosis indicating necrotizing vasculitis is rarely seen.[2,4–5] Histopathology of PLC lesions usually shows a perivascular chronic inflammatory cell infiltrate in the superficial dermis, focal disappearance

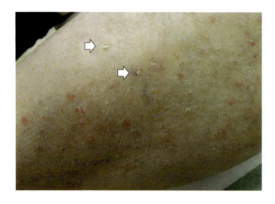

FIGURE 19.2 Pityriasis lichenoides chronica: several reddish-brownish papules, some of which presenting a characteristic centrally adherent micaceous scale (arrows).

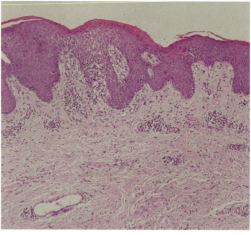

FIGURE 19.3 Histopathology of pityriasis lichenoides chronica: perivascular chronic inflammatory cell infiltrate in the superficial dermis, focal disappearance of the dermal-epidermal interface, focal parakeratosis, acanthosis, lymphocytic exocytosis, and some extravasated erythrocytes (H&E ×100).

of the dermal-epidermal interface, focal parakeratosis, slight acanthosis, and preservation of the granular layer (Figure 19.3). Spongiosis and extravasated erythrocytes are often present but are usually not marked. Necrosis and ballooning of keratinocytes are typically missing or minimal.[2,5]

DERMATOSCOPY/ VIDEODERMATOSCOPY FEATURES

Only one investigation of PLEVA exists.[6] It was performed on two patients and revealed (at ×20 magnification) in both cases the presence of papules with a central whitish patch or crusted lesions with an amorphous brownish structure, both surrounded by a well-defined ring of pinpoint and/or linear vascular structures with a targetoid aspect (Figure 19.4). At higher magnification, the vessels appeared dilated and convoluted, with some of them showing a glomerular pattern or linear arrangement. Moreover, non-blanchable reddish globules were observed in all fields (Figure 19.5). Such aspects correlated with the presence of dilation and engorgement of blood vessels and microhemorrhages in the papillary dermis[6] (Figure 19.6). The above-described dermatoscopic features are indicative

Inflammatory Diseases

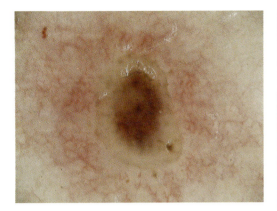

FIGURE 19.4 Dermatoscopy of a papule of PLEVA: presence of a central amorphous brownish structure surrounded by a well-defined ring of vascular structures configuring a targetoid appearance (×20).

of PLEVA and may help in the differential diagnosis from other similar skin eruptions, mainly including chickenpox, arthropod bites, leukocytoclastic vasculitis, and, particularly, lymphomatoid papulosis in its early and late stages.[1–3,7] In a dermatoscopic study of eight cases of lymphomatoid papulosis, the initial inflammatory papules were characterized by a vascular pattern of tortuous irregular vessels, surrounded by white structureless areas, radiating from the center to the periphery of the lesion. As the disease progressed to late necrotic lesions, such characteristic vascular pattern was detectable

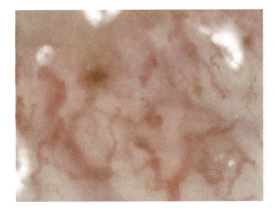

FIGURE 19.5 Dermatoscopy of a papule of PLEVA: at higher magnification (×300), the vessels appear dilated and convoluted, with some of them showing a glomerular pattern or linear arrangement.

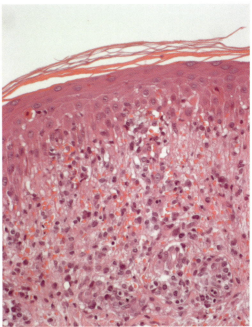

FIGURE 19.6 Histopathology of PLEVA: presence of dilation and engorgement of blood vessels and micro-hemorrhages in papillary dermis.

only at the periphery, while the center of the lesions showed a brown-gray structureless area.[7]

Regarding PLC, a retrospective analysis of eight patients[8] found that orange-yellowish structureless areas, likely reflecting extravasated erythrocytes and consequent hemosiderin degradation products, and nondotted vessels (including milky-red areas/globules, linear irregular and branching vessels), corresponding to dilatation of superficial dermal vessels (Figure 19.7), were the most frequent dermatoscopic findings being present in seven cases. Considering the specific pattern of nondotted vessels, linear irregular vessels, branching vessels, and milky-red areas/globules were present in six, four, and two patients, respectively. Other observed dermatoscopic findings were focally distributed dotted vessels (present in five cases) and hypopigmented areas (evident in one patient only). The latter feature is probably more typical of late lesions, which often leave postinflammatory hypopigmentation.[1–3] Dermatoscopy may assist in the clinical diagnosis of PLC and may facilitate its differentiation from other papulosquamous dermatoses, such as lichen

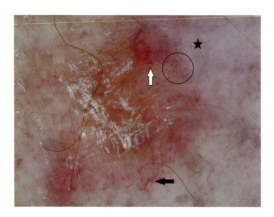 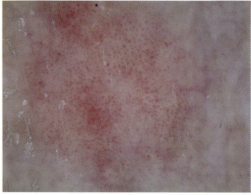

FIGURE 19.7 Dermatoscopy of a papule of pityriasis lichenoides chronica: orange-yellowish structureless areas in the center of the lesion and focally distributed dotted (black circle), linear irregular (white arrow), and branching vessels (black arrow) at the periphery. Hypopigmented areas (the lighter areas of the surrounding healthy skin) are also evident (black star) (×10).

FIGURE 19.8 Dermatoscopy of guttate psoriasis: monomorphic dotted vessels distributed in a diffuse pattern (×10).

planus, distinguished by the presence of whitish crossing lines (Wickham striae); pityriasis rosea, which often shows peripheral scales and focally distributed dotted vessels on a yellowish background;[9] and guttate psoriasis. The latter typically shows a distinct monomorphic picture quite similar to that commonly found in plaque psoriasis,[8,10–11] with dotted vessels distributed in a diffuse pattern (Figure 19.8). Besides the above-mentioned disorders, in some instances PLC must be differentiated from the mature stage of lymphomatoid papulosis, as described earlier.

In conclusion, dermatoscopy may improve the clinical diagnosis of both PLEVA and PLC and also may be useful for the differential diagnosis with other clinically similar dermatoses and between themselves. In fact, although both PLEVA and PLC belong to the same spectrum of disease, they present different dermatoscopic features due to their different underlying histological findings.

REFERENCES

1. Whittaker SJ. Cutaneous lymphomas and lymphocytic infiltrates. In: *Rook's Textbook of Dermatology*. 8th ed. Burns T, Breathnach S, Cox N, Griffiths C, eds. Oxford: Wiley-Blackwell, 2010:57:54–57.
2. Bowers S, Warshaw EM. Pityriasis lichenoides and its subtypes. *J Am Acad Dermatol*. 2006;55:557–72.
3. Wood GS, Hu CH, Liu R. Parapsoriasis and pityriasis lichenoides. In: *Fitzpatrick's Dermatology in General Medicine*. 8th ed. Goldsmith LA, Katz SI, Gilchrest BA, Paller AS, Leffell DJ, Wolff K, eds. New York: McGraw-Hill, 2012:291–96.
4. Fernandes NF, Rozdeba PJ, Schwartz RA, et al. Pityriasis lichenoides et varioliformis acuta: A disease spectrum. *Int J Dermatol*. 2010;49:257–61.
5. Wang WL, Lazar A. Lichenoid and interface dermatitis. In: *McKee's Pathology of the Skin*. 4th ed. Calonje JE, Brenn T, Lazar AJF, McKee PH, eds. Philadelphia: Elsevier Saunders, 2012:255–58.
6. Lacarrubba F, Micali G. Dermoscopy of pityriasis lichenoides et varioliformis acuta. *Arch Dermatol*. 2010;146:1322.
7. Moura FN, Thomas L, Balme B, Dalle S. Dermoscopy of lymphomatoid Papulosis. *Arch Dermatol*. 2009;145:966–67.

8. Errichetti E, Lacarrubba F, Micali G, et al. Differentiation of pityriasis lichenoides chronica from guttate psoriasis by dermoscopy. *Clin Exp Dermatol*. 2015;40:804–6.
9. Lallas A, Kyrgidis A, Tzellos TG, et al. Accuracy of dermoscopic criteria for the diagnosis of psoriasis, dermatitis, lichen planus and pityriasis rosea. *Br J Dermatol*. 2012;166:1198–205.
10. Stinco G, Buligan C, Errichetti E, et al. Clinical and capillaroscopic modifications of the psoriatic plaque during therapy: Observations with oral acitretin. *Dermatol Res Pract*. 2013;2013:781942.
11. Lallas A, Apalla Z, Tzellos T, Lefaki I. Photoletter to the editor: Dermoscopy in clinically atypical psoriasis. *J Dermatol Case Rep*. 2012;6:61–62.

20 Inflammatory diseases
Granulomatous skin disorders and Wolf's isotopic response lesions

Francisco Vázquez-López, Celia Gómez de Castro, and Noemi Eiris-Salvado

GRANULOMATOUS SKIN DISORDERS

DEFINITION

The term *granulomatous skin disorders* (GSDs) encompasses a variety of infectious and noninfectious conditions characterized by an inflammatory granulomatous infiltrate. They differ in their pathogenesis as well as in their clinical and histopathologic presentation.

EPIDEMIOLOGY/ETIOPATHOGENESIS

The prevalence of GSDs is unknown. Granulomatous reactions develop as a chronic immune response to an immunogenic agent that cannot be eliminated or is only slowly degraded by the immune system. The inciting antigen can be infectious and noninfectious.

CLINICAL PRESENTATION/DIAGNOSIS

The clinical spectrum of GSDs is various, including cutaneous sarcoidosis (CS), lupus vulgaris (LV), cutaneous leishmaniasis (CL), granulomatous rosacea (GR), granuloma annulare (GA), or necrobiosis lipoidica (NL). The diagnosis is generally histopathological: GSDs are characterized by an inflammatory infiltrate with epithelioid or giant cells. An infiltrate may be considered granulomatous if it consists of at least 50% of histiocytes/macrophages (Figure 20.1).

DERMATOSCOPY/VIDEODERMATOSCOPY FEATURES

Dermatoscopic semiology of GSDs is based on recognition of the morphology, color, and arrangement of different vascular, nonvascular, and follicular structures such as yellow patches (YPs), arboriform or short linear and dotted vessels, milia-like cysts, and follicular plugs. Different dermatoscopic findings have been reported for CS, LV, CL, GR, GA, and NL.[1–12]

The translucent, round/oval orange YPs represent the main dermatoscopic finding[13] of GSDs (Figures 20.2–20.5): although not predictive for a specific disease, it is highly suggestive of an underlying dermal granuloma. YPs may appear as individual, granular, yellowish nodules ("grains of sand") (Figure 20.3) or yellowish-brown, homogeneous discoloration ("apple-jelly" sign) (Figure 20.4). Linear or branching vessels are common additional dermatoscopic findings that may obscure YPs. In such cases, blanching the lesions (with diascopy or contact dermatoscopy) improves their recognition. In the authors' experience, diascopy may reveal a

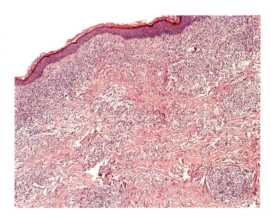

FIGURE 20.1 Histopathology of a noninfectious granulomatous skin disorder (sarcoidal skin lesion with nude dermal granulomas).

FIGURE 20.2 Dermatoscopy of a granulomatous skin lesion showing yellow patches (translucent, round/oval orange-yellowish areas) (×10).

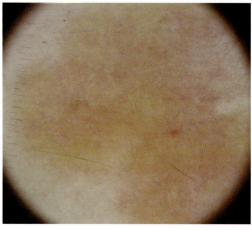

FIGURE 20.4 Dermatoscopy of homogeneous yellow patches ("apple-jelly" sign), which may appear in different granulomatous skin disorders (×10).

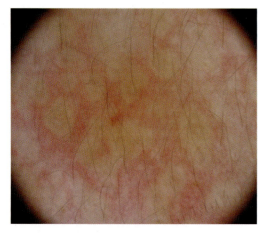

FIGURE 20.3 Dermatoscopy of granular ("grains of sand") yellow patches, which may appear in different granulomatous skin disorders (×10).

similar pattern despite being without magnification.[12] The dermatoscopic detection of YPs is suggestive of the diagnosis of a GSD. However, a biopsy should be performed to confirm it and to differentiate among different GSDs.

Arborizing linear vessels are a constant finding in NL but are rare in GA and CS. At dermatoscopy, NL is typified by a prominent network of branching arborizing vessels within a yellow background color either alone or in combination with white or red areas[6–8] (Figure 20.6). Ulcerations and yellow crusts represent the most common additional features.[8] GA shows heterogeneous dermatoscopic findings. Vessels of GA are generally dotted or short linear and rarely linear arborizing. The background color

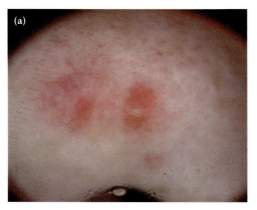
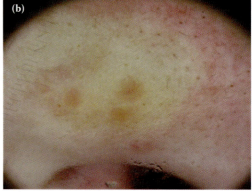

FIGURE 20.5 Dermatoscopy of a granulomatous skin disorder. (a) Yellow patches may be obscured by vessels if they are prominent. (b) Blanching them with diascopy is necessary for revealing yellow patches in deeply red lesions (×10).

Inflammatory Diseases

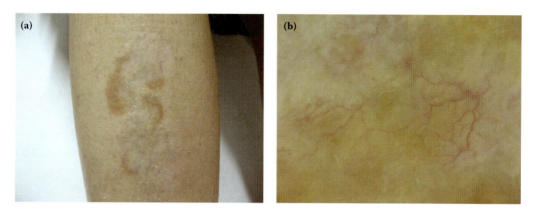

FIGURE 20.6 (a) Typical lesions of necrobiosis lipoidica on a leg. (b) Dermatoscopy showing the presence of arborizing vessels within yellow patches (×10).

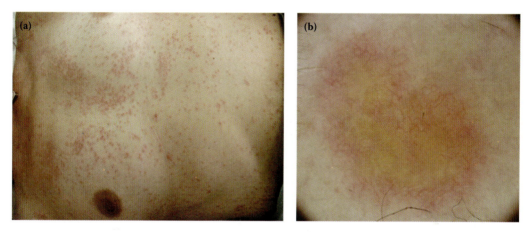

FIGURE 20.7 (a) Lichenoid sarcoidosis of the trunk. (b) Dermatoscopy showing the presence of yellow patches and the absence of Wickham striae (×10).

varies from white to red. CL may show a wider range of changes (including follicular plugs, "yellow tears," hyperkeratosis, erosion/ulceration, "white starburst-like pattern," salmon-colored ovoid structures) and variable vessels (comma-shaped, linear, dotted, polymorphous, hairpin, arborizing, corkscrew, and glomerular-like vessels).[9–11] It has been suggested that in geographical areas in which CL is common, dermatoscopy may be a useful, practical, and noninvasive diagnostic tool.[11] Dermatoscopy may be useful for discriminating between lichenoid sarcoidosis and lichen planus, by revealing the YPs of the former (Figure 20.7) in contrast to the pathognomonic white Wickham striae of the latter[13–14] (Figure 20.8).

Finally, dermatoscopy may be useful for the monitoring of some GSD. For example, it may

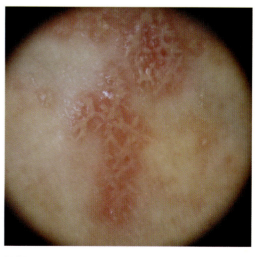

FIGURE 20.8 Dermatoscopy of lichen planus: presence of the pathognomonic Wickham striae (×10).

reveal small, scarcely evident erosions in NL, which may herald deterioration of the disease (i.e., the development of clinically apparent ulceration).[8]

WOLF'S ISOTOPIC RESPONSE LESIONS

Definition

The development of an unrelated (secondary) cutaneous disorder over the exact site of a previous (primary) healed skin disease is known as *Wolf's isotopic response* (WIR).[12,15–16]

Epidemiology/Etiopathogenesis

WIR is frequently, but not exclusively, post-herpetic. Post-herpetic WIR, which is mainly secondary to varicella-zoster virus infection, is often underdiagnosed due to its rarity and the broad spectrum of clinical and histopathological presentations. Among them, granulomatous reactions are the most frequent (tuberculoid, sarcoidal, unclassified granulomatous dermatitis or granuloma annulare).[16]

The pathological mechanisms of WIR are still unknown, although local neuro-immune alterations, delayed-type hypersensitivity reaction, and immune dysfunction (usually related to hematological malignancy or immunosuppressive therapy) might contribute to its development.[12]

Clinical presentation/Diagnosis

WIR is rare and may be easily misdiagnosed. A precise history denoting a previous and different disorder on the same area of WIR can lead the dermatologist to suspect it.

Dermatoscopy/Videodermatoscopy features

Dermatoscopy can be applied for differentiating between the various skin diseases causing WIR, by revealing differential dermatoscopic patterns (Table 20.1).[12] It should be noted that dermatoscopic findings may be specific or "unspecific." Unspecific features may be rendered valuable when coupled with certain other clinical and dermatoscopic criteria, forming a set of features that leads to either a single diagnosis or a narrowed list of differential diagnoses. Evaluation of positive and negative findings (e.g., presence/absence of YPs, Wickham striae, rainbow pattern, etc.) improves the clinical interpretation of WIR lesions. Dermatoscopic detection in these lesions of granular or homogeneous YPs with a variable hue (orange, whitish, brown) is considered suggestive of a granulomatous etiology

TABLE 20.1
Differential dermatoscopic patterns in post-herpetic WIR lesions

Secondary isotopic skin disease	Dermatoscopic pattern
Inflammatory dermatoses	
Sarcoidosis	Orange-yellowish areas, linear vessels
Granuloma annulare	Variable (vessels and background color)
Lichen planus	Wickham striae, mixed vessels
Psoriasis	Dotted vessels with regular distribution
Lichen sclerosus et atrophicus	White areas, keratotic plugs
Rosacea	Polygonal vessels
Malignant tumors	
Kaposi's sarcoma	"Rainbow pattern," red-blue lacunar areas, purple-brownish areas
Basal cell carcinoma	Arborizing vessels, leaf-like areas, large blue-gray ovoid nests, multiple blue-gray globules, spoke wheel areas, ulceration
Other (breast cancer, angiosarcoma)	Variable
Infections (bacterial, fungal, viral)	Variable

Inflammatory Diseases

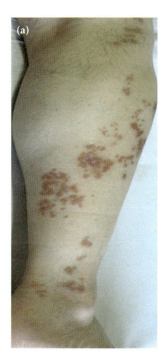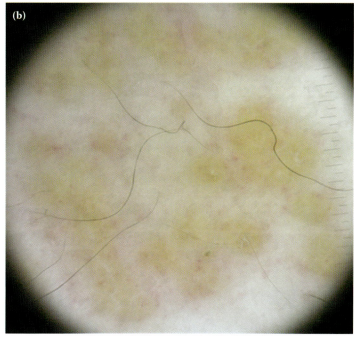

FIGURE 20.9 (a) Post-herpetic Wolf's isotopic response of the right leg. (b) Dermatoscopy showing the presence of yellow patches (×10).

(Figure 20.9); recognition of other characteristic features (e.g., Wickham striae) may orientate the clinician toward another diagnosis, such as lichen planus.

REFERENCES

1. Brasiello M, Zalaudek I, Ferrara G, et al. Lupus vulgaris: A new look at an old symptom—The lupoma observed with dermoscopy. *Dermatology.* 2009;218:172–74.
2. Lallas A, Argenziano G, Apalla Z, et al. Dermoscopic patterns of common facial inflammatory skin diseases. *J Eur Acad Dermatol Venereol.* 2014;28:609–14.
3. Pellicano R, Tiodorovic-Zivkovic D, Gourhant J-Y, et al. Dermoscopy of cutaneous sarcoidosis. *Dermatology.* 2010;221:51–54.
4. Vázquez-López F, Palacios-Garcia L, Gomez-Diez S, et al. Dermoscopy for discriminating between lichenoid sarcoidosis and lichen planus. *Arch Dermatol.* 2011;147:1130.
5. Balestri R, La Placa M, Bardazzi F, Rech G. Dermoscopic subpatterns of granulomatous skin diseases. *J Am Acad Dermatol.* 2013;69:e217–18.
6. Pellicano R, Caldarola G, Filabozzi P, et al. Dermoscopy of necrobiosis lipoidica and granuloma annulare. *Dermatology.* 2013;226:319–23.
7. Lallas A, Zaballos P, Zalaudek I, et al. Dermoscopic patterns of granuloma annulare and necrobiosis lipoidica. *Clin Exp Dermatol.* 2013;38:425–27.
8. Bakos RM, Cartell A, Bakos L. Dermatoscopy of early-onset necrobiosis lipoidica. *J Am Acad Dermatol.* 2012;66:e143–44.
9. Llambrich A, Zaballos P, Terrasa F, et al. Dermoscopy of cutaneous leishmaniasis. *Br J Dermatol.* 2009;160:756–61.
10. Taheri AR, Pishgooei N, Maleki M, et al. Dermoscopic features of cutaneous leishmaniasis. *Int J Dermatol.* 2013;52:1361–66.
11. Yucel A, Gunasti S, Denli Y, Uzun S. Cutaneous leishmaniasis: New dermoscopic findings. *Int J Dermatol.* 2013;52:831–37.
12. Eirís N, Vázquez-López F, Palacios-García L, et al. Value of dermoscopy for the differential diagnosis of Wolf's post herpetic isotopic response. *Australas J Dermatol.* 2015;56(1):29–31.
13. Lallas A, Giacomel J, Argenziano G, et al. Dermoscopy in general dermatology: Practical tips for the clinician. *Br J Dermatol.* 2014;170:514–26.

14. Pan Y, Chamberlain AJ, Bailey M, et al. Dermatoscopy aids in the diagnosis of the solitary red scaly patch or plaque-features distinguishing superficial basal cell carcinoma, intraepidermal carcinoma, and psoriasis. *J Am Acad Dermatol.* 2008;59:268–74.
15. Wolf R, Wolf D, Ruocco E, et al. Wolf's isotopic response. *Clin Dermatol.* 2011;29:237–40.
16. Requena L, Kutzner H, Escalonilla P, et al. Cutaneous reactions at sites of herpes zoster scars: An expanded spectrum. *Br J Dermatol.* 1998;138:161.

21 Nonpigmented skin lesions
Clear cell acanthoma

Francesco Lacarrubba, Federica Dall'Oglio, and Giuseppe Micali

DEFINITION

Clear cell acanthoma (CCA) is a usually solitary benign epidermal tumor first described by Degos in 1962.[1]

EPIDEMIOLOGY/ETIOPATHOGENESIS

The mean age of onset is about 52 years, with equal frequency in men and women.[2–5] CCA occurs frequently on the lower extremities, but other anatomic sites (trunk, upper extremities) have been reported. Multiple lesions (from 2 to 400) are rarely encountered; the rate between solitary and multiple CCA is estimated to be 1:9–1:15.[2–6] Ichthyosis and varicose veins are the most frequent associated findings. The etiology is not well understood. Although some authors suggest that the lesion may represent a benign epithelial neoplasm, others consider the disease as a localized reactive inflammatory dermatosis (pseudotumor).[2–5]

CLINICAL PRESENTATION/DIAGNOSIS

CCA clinically appears as a dome-shaped, sharply circumscribed, reddish papule, variable in size from 5–20 mm. A peripheral scaling collarette is characteristic but not always present (Figures 21.1 and 21.2).

The differential diagnosis of single and/or multiple CCA includes several conditions, such as histiocytomas, seborrheic keratoses, basal cell carcinomas, pyogenic granulomas, syringomas, hidradenomas, leiomyomas, fibromas, perifolliculomas, disseminated granuloma annulare, lichen planus, and sarcoidosis. The diagnosis of CCA is usually confirmed by histologic examination, showing acanthosis, papillomatosis, and a sharply demarcated epidermal proliferation of keratinocytes with a clear and slightly larger cytoplasm, with a positive periodic acid–Schiff (PAS) stain. In the superficial dermis, enlarged capillaries in the papillae are evident.

DERMATOSCOPY/VIDEODERMATOSCOPY FEATURES

In 2001 Blum and colleagues, reporting a single case of CCA, first described a characteristic dermatoscopic vascular pattern at ×20 magnification, consisting of "partly homogeneous, symmetrically or bunch-like arranged, pinpoint-like capillaries."[7] Although the authors stated that a similar pattern could also be seen in psoriatic plaques after removal of the scales, they concluded that dermatoscopy might be helpful to differentiate CCA from other skin tumors.[7]

Bugatti and colleagues reported six cases of CCA characterized by this psoriasis-like vascular finding on dermatoscopy.[8] They observed that the dotted vessels were regularly distributed in a reticular array; they also detected the presence of a squamous surface with translucid collarette as an additional characteristic finding. The authors concluded that the psoriasis-like pattern of CCA would appear to provide further evidence of a neoangiogenetic inflammatory process rather than a neoplastic one for CCA formation.[8]

Zalaudek and colleagues stated that dermatoscopic features of CCA are different from those of psoriasis[9] as, in their experience, in CCA the dotted vessels are linearly arranged as pearls on a line, whereas in psoriasis they are homogeneously and regularly distributed throughout the entire lesion. Therefore, in

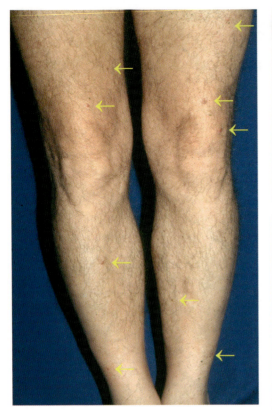

FIGURE 21.1 Multiple clear cell acanthomas of the legs (arrows).

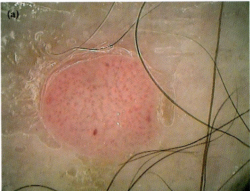

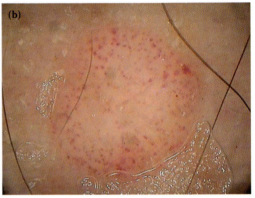

FIGURES 21.3 (a–b) Dermatoscopy of clear cell acanthomas: symmetrical and homogeneous pinpoint-like vascular structures with a pearl-like disposition (×30).

their opinion, these pearl-like vessels represent a peculiar pattern of CCA.[9]

In the same year the authors of this chapter studied the dermatoscopic pattern of multiple CCAs in a single patient,[10] with all of them showing the same pattern, that is, symmetrical and homogeneous pinpoint-like vascular structures throughout the entire lesion. The pearl-like vessels' disposition, at least in a portion of each lesion, was always present (Figure 21.3), while the presence of a net-like pattern was a frequent but not constant finding (Figure 21.4). At higher magnification (×200) each vascular structure appeared to have a bush-like aspect (Figure 21.5).

The dermatoscopic pattern of CCA, which has been successively confirmed by other reports,[11–13] corresponds to the histologic aspect of regularly elongated rete ridges and enlarged capillaries in the dermal papillae (Figure 21.6). For this reason, it resembles that of psoriasis and, possibly, of other psoriasiform disorders (such as pityriasis rubra pilaris and some variants of contact dermatitis) characterized by epidermal proliferation and dermal capillaries dilatation,

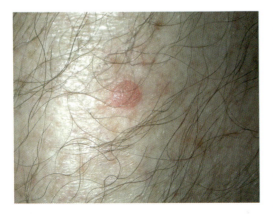

FIGURE 21.2 Close-up clinical view of a clear cell acanthoma: reddish, sharply circumscribed papule with a peripheral scaling collarette.

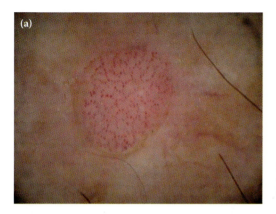

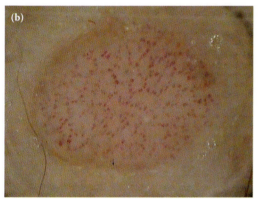

FIGURES 21.4 (a–b) Dermatoscopy of clear cell acanthomas: symmetrical and homogeneous pinpoint-like vascular structures arranged in a net-like pattern (×30).

thus implying the need for additional diagnostic criteria. Differential diagnosis from psoriasis is particularly relevant in the case of multiple

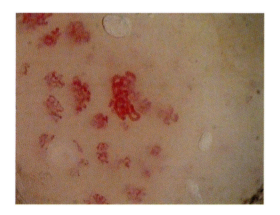

FIGURE 21.5 High-magnification videodermatoscopy of clear cell acanthoma depicting the bush-like aspect of pinpoint-like capillaries (×200).

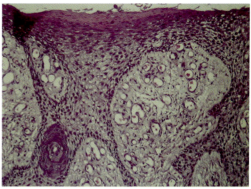

FIGURE 21.6 Histopathology of clear cell acanthoma showing regularly elongated rete ridges and enlarged capillaries in the dermal papillae.

CCAs. Other cutaneous conditions, such as warts, actinic and seborrheic keratoses, Bowen's disease, squamous cell carcinoma, hypopigmented Spitz nevus, melanoma, and melanoma metastasis may sometimes show pinpoint-like vessels. In these instances, however, a correct evaluation of anamnestic and clinical features along with additional dermatoscopic features will help to address the correct diagnosis.

In conclusion, dermatoscopy may improve the clinical diagnosis of single or multiple CCAs, ruling out clinically similar disorders that do not show the same features of CCA.

REFERENCES

1. Degos R, Delort J, Civatte J, Baptista P. Tumeur épidermique d'aspect particulier: Acanthome à cellules claires. *Ann Dermatol Syphiligr.* 1962:89;361–71.
2. Trau H, Fisher BK, Schewach-Millet M. Multiple clear cell acanthomas. *Arch Dermatol.* 1980;116:433–34.
3. Bonnetblanc JM, Delrous JL, Catanzano G, et al. Multiple clear cell acanthoma. *Arch Dermatol.* 1981;117:1.
4. Innocenzi D, Barduagni F, Cerio R, Wolter M. Disseminated eruptive clear cell acanthoma: A case report with review of the literature. *Clin Exp Dermatol.* 1994;19:249–53.
5. Wilde JL, Meffert JJ, McCollough ML. Polypoid clear cell acanthoma of the scalp. *Cutis.* 2001;67:149–51.
6. Burg G, Wursch TH, Fah J, Elsner P. Eruptive hamartomatous clear-cell acanthomas. *Dermatology.* 1994;189:437-9.

7. Blum A, Metzler G, Bauer J, et al. The dermatoscopic pattern of clear cell acanthoma resembles psoriasis vulgaris. *Dermatology.* 2001;203:50–52.
8. Bugatti L, Filosa G, Broganelli P, Tomasini C. Psoriasis-like dermoscopic pattern of clear cell acanthoma. *J Eur Acad Dermatol Venereol.* 2003;17:452–55.
9. Zalaudek I, Hofmann-Wellenhof R, Argenziano G. Dermoscopy of clear-cell acanthoma differs from dermoscopy of psoriasis. *Dermatology.* 2003;207:428.
10. Lacarrubba F, De Pasquale R, Micali G. Videodermatoscopy improves the clinical diagnostic accuracy of multiple clear cell acanthoma. *Eur J Dermatol.* 2003;13:596–98.
11. Akin FY, Ertam I, Ceylan C, et al. Clear cell acanthoma: New observations on dermatoscopy. *Indian J Dermatol Venereol Leprol.* 2008;74:285–87.
12. Ardigo M, Buffon RB, Scope A, et al. Comparing in vivo reflectance confocal microscopy, dermoscopy, and histology of clear-cell acanthoma. *Dermatol Surg.* 2009;35:952–59.
13. Betti R, Menni S, Cerri A, Crosti C. A reddish papular lesion on the scrotum: A quiz. *Acta Derm Venereol.* 2011;91:211–12.

22 Nonpigmented skin lesions
Pyogenic granuloma

Pedro Zaballos Diego

DEFINITION

Pyogenic granuloma (PG) is a relatively common benign vascular lesion of the skin and mucous membranes. This misnamed entity is neither infectious nor granulomatous, and therefore some authors prefer the term *lobular capillary hemangioma* to describe these lesions because of the histologic findings.

EPIDEMIOLOGY/ETIOPATHOGENESIS

PG is relatively common, and it is especially frequent in children and young adults.[1-3] It represents 0.5% of all skin nodules in children.[4] The exact etiopathogenesis of this condition is unknown. It has been thought to be a reactive hyperproliferative vascular response to a variety of stimuli, such as infective organisms, penetrating injury, hormonal factors, and retinoid therapy. PG usually develops at the site of a preexisting injury, where it evolves rapidly over a period of weeks to a maximum size and then shrinks in a fibroma that can regress within a few months. A few reports of lesions developing in a preexisting nevus flammeus or spider angioma exist.

CLINICAL PRESENTATION/DIAGNOSIS

The typical lesion appears as a papule or polypoid lesion with a glistening surface, which bleeds easily. Sites of predilection include the gingiva, lips, face, mucosa of the nose, and the extremities (mainly the fingers). PG with satellitosis, a subcutaneous subtype, an intravenous subtype, and a disseminated variant have been described. The gingival lesion developed during pregnancy and known as epulis gravidorum is considered a variant of this tumor.

Although the clinical diagnosis of PG is rather easy, in some instances the differentiation from other benign and malignant tumors, such as amelanotic melanoma, is difficult to determine. In 38% of one case series,[5] the clinical diagnosis of PG proved to be wrong. Misdiagnoses documented in medical literature mainly include keratoacanthoma, squamous cell carcinoma, basal cell carcinoma, inflamed seborrhoeic keratosis, common warts, melanocytic nevus, Spitz nevus, amelanotic melanoma, metastasic carcinoma, Kaposi's sarcoma, and true hemangiomas.[1-6]

The histopathologic findings in all variants of PG are similar. Early lesions resemble granulation tissue that consists of numerous capillaries and venules with plump endothelial cells arrayed radially toward the skin surface (usually eroded, ulcerated, and covered with scabs) amid an edematous stroma containing a mixed inflammatory infiltrate. The matured polypoid lesion exhibits a fibromyxoid stroma separating the lesion into a lobular pattern. Each lobule is composed of aggregations of capillaries and venules with plump endothelial cells. In this stage, reepithelialization of the surface and a peripheral collarette of hyperplastic adnexal epithelium may be noted, with less inflammatory infiltrate. Older lesions tend to organize and, in time, PG resolves into fibroma.[1-4]

DERMATOSCOPY/VIDEODERMATOSCOPY FEATURES

Dermatoscopy may be helpful in the recognition of PG.[7-9] The results of one study of 122 PGs reveal that five structures are basically associated with this lesion: a reddish homogeneous area (RHA), white collarette (WC), "white rail lines" (WRL) that intersect the lesion, vascular structures (VS), and ulceration.[9]

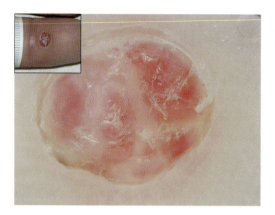

FIGURE 22.1 Dermatoscopy of pyogenic granuloma: reddish homogeneous area with white rail lines that intersect the lesion surrounded by a white collarette. Superficial scales can also be observed (×10).

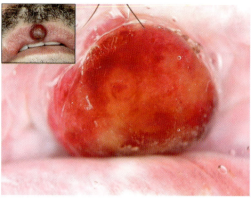

FIGURE 22.3 Dermatoscopy of pyogenic granuloma located on the upper lip: reddish homogeneous area surrounded by a white collarette (×10).

The RHA is a homogeneous zone, whose color varies from completely red to red with whitish zones, which is present in the majority of the lesion and histologically corresponds to the presence of numerous small capillaries or proliferating vessels that are set in a myxoid stroma (Figures 22.1–22.7). RHA exhibited a high sensitivity for PG (96.7%) but low specificity because it is commonly found in other tumors, especially in amelanotic melanomas (Figure 22.8).[9]

The WC is a ring-shaped or arquate squamous structure that is usually located at the periphery of the lesion and corresponds to the hyperplastic adnexal epithelium that partially or totally embraces the lesion at the periphery of most PGs (Figures 22.1–22.3, 22.5, and 22.7). WC demonstrated to be the most specific structure for PG, with 90.7% specificity, although it may be also observed in clear cell acanthomas, basal cell carcinomas, Kaposi's sarcomas, solitary angiokeratomas, and even amelanotic melanomas.[9]

The WRLs are defined as whitish streaks or bands that intersect the PG and histologically correspond to the fibrous septa that surround the capillary tufts or lobules in more advanced cases (Figures 22.1 and 22.4). WRLs exhibit a

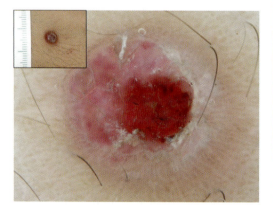

FIGURE 22.2 Dermatoscopy of pyogenic granuloma: reddish homogeneous area surrounded by a white collarette. Scales and ulceration can also be observed (×10).

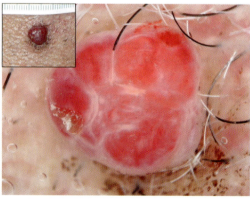

FIGURE 22.4 Dermatoscopy of pyogenic granuloma: reddish homogeneous area and white rail lines that intersect the lesion. This is a pedunculated lesion and, in these cases, it is difficult to see the white collarette on polarized contact dermatoscopy. A scale in the left part of the lesion and an area of ulceration in the upper part can also be observed (×10).

Nonpigmented Skin Lesions

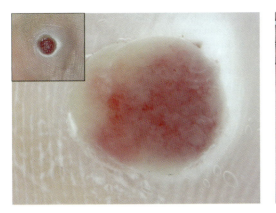

FIGURE 22.5 Dermatoscopy of pyogenic granuloma: reddish homogeneous area surrounded by a white collarette; several vascular structures can also be observed. In these cases, it is mandatory to remove the lesions to avoid misdiagnosing an amelanotic melanoma (×10).

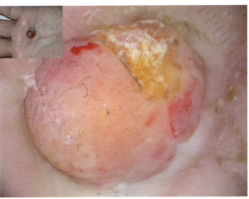

FIGURE 22.7 Dermatoscopy of pyogenic granuloma: reddish homogeneous area with vascular structures and ulceration surrounded by a white collarette (×10).

good specificity (81.4%), but they can also be observed in dermatofibromas, basal cell carcinomas, melanomas, and other vascular tumors.[9]

Areas of ulceration (Figures 22.2, 22.4–22.7) and VS (Figures 22.5–22.7) have been detected in 45.9% and 45.1% of PGs, respectively, but both features exhibited low sensitivity and specificity. VS may be composed of different types of vessels: dotted vessels, hairpin vessels, telangiectasias, linear-irregular vessels, and polymorphous atypical vessels.[9]

None of the dermatoscopic structures evaluated in the study demonstrated to be 100% specific for PG as an isolated criterion.[9] Consequently, seven exclusive patterns were made up from the combination of RHA, WC, WRL, and VS to find a possible specific pattern associated with PG. Three patterns (RHA+WC+WRL, RHA+WC, and RHA+WC+WRL+VS) were not found in any amelanotic/hypomelanotic melanomas; however, melanomas with all of these structures as an isolated criterion may be found, so a melanoma could theoretically display these patterns.[9]

In conclusion, dermatoscopy has been shown to be a useful tool to evaluate PG, but

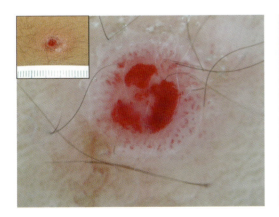

FIGURE 22.6 Dermatoscopy of pyogenic granuloma: central area of ulceration and polymorphous/atypical vessels (linear irregular, hairpin, and glomerular vessels). The lesion should be excised to avoid misdiagnosing an amelanotic melanoma (×10).

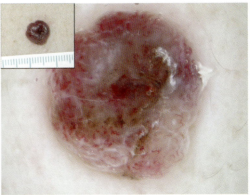

FIGURE 22.8 Dermatoscopy of amelanotic melanoma previously clinically diagnosed as PG: reddish homogeneous area, polymorphous/atypical vessels, white lines that do not intersect the lesion (chrysalis), and remnants of pigment can be observed (×10).

it is advisable to remove PGs to perform a histopathologic evaluation as they continue to be a dangerous simulator of amelanotic melanoma by clinical and dermatoscopic examination (Figure 22.8).

REFERENCES

1. Mooney MA, Janninger CK. Pyogenic granuloma. *Cutis*. 1995;55:133–36.
2. Pagliai KA, Cohen BA. Pyogenic granuloma in children. *Pediatr Dermatol*. 2004;21:10–13.
3. Requena L, Sangueza OP. Cutaneous vascular proliferation. Part II. Hyperplasias and benign neoplasms. *J Am Acad Dermatol*. 1997;37:887–919.
4. Grimalt R, Caputo R. Symmetric pyogenic granuloma. *J Am Acad Dermatol*. 1993;29:652.
5. Rowe L. Granuloma pyogenicum. *AMA Arch Dermatol*. 1958;78:341–47.
6. Elmets CA, Ceilley RI. Amelanotic melanoma presenting as a pyogenic granuloma. *Cutis*. 1980;25:164–67.
7. Zaballos P, Llambrich A, Cuellar F, et al. Dermoscopic findings in pyogenic granuloma. *Br J Dermatol*. 2006;154:1108–11.
8. Zaballos P, Salsench E, Puig S, Malvehy J. Dermoscopy of pyogenic granulomas. *Arch Dermatol*. 2007;143:824.
9. Zaballos P, Carulla M, Ozdemir F, et al. Dermoscopy of pyogenic granuloma: A morphological study. *Br J Dermatol*. 2010;163:1229–37.

23 Nonpigmented skin lesions
Angiokeratoma

Anna Elisa Verzì, Francesco Lacarrubba, and Giuseppe Micali

DEFINITION

Angiokeratoma is a benign hyperkeratotic vascular proliferation.

EPIDEMIOLOGY/ETIOPATHOGENESIS

The prevalence of angiokeratomas, which are more frequent in men, is estimated to be approximately 0.16% among the general population.[1] The exact etiology is unknown; pregnancy, chilblains, trauma, and tissue asphyxia are hypothesized as causal factors. Congenital cases have been reported.[2]

CLINICAL PRESENTATION/DIAGNOSIS

Clinically, angiokeratoma appears as a solitary or multiple deep red to blue-black hyperkeratotic papule with a diameter ranging from 2–10 mm (Figures 23.1a and 23.2a). It is usually asymptomatic, although some patients may report mild to moderate pain and bleeding following irritation or trauma. Five clinical variants are recognized: *angiokeratoma corporis diffusum*, localized over the trunk and proximal extremities and associated with Fabry's disease; *angiokeratoma of Mibelli*, usually on the hands and feet; *angiokeratoma of Fordyce*, limited to the scrotum; *angiokeratoma circumscriptum*, which appears at birth in a unilaterally zosteriform shape and may later become large and warty; and *solitary and multiple angiokeratomas*, the most common variant, similar to Mibelli type, localized on the whole body but more frequently on the lower extremities.[2–3]

Histologically, angiokeratoma shows dilated subepidermal congested vessels and large lacunae in the papillary dermis containing erythrocytes or thrombi. The epidermis shows acanthosis, papillomatosis, and hyperkeratosis; there is no involvement of the deep dermis and hypodermis.[2,4–5]

DERMATOSCOPY/VIDEODERMATOSCOPY FEATURES

Dermatoscopic features of angiokeratoma are represented by a spectrum of signs including red lacunae, dark lacunae, whitish veil, erythema, and hemorrhagic crusts (Figures 23.1b, 23.2b).[1,4–6] Red lacunae appear as sharply ovoid/roundish red or red-blue structures corresponding to wide dilated vascular spaces located in the upper or middle dermis. Dark lacunae are the most peculiar features; they appear as sharply ovoid/round dark blue to black areas and represent dilated vascular spaces in the upper dermis partially or completely thrombosed. Whitish veil refers to an ill-defined structureless area with an overlying whitish "ground-glass" film due to hyperkeratosis and acanthosis. Erythema and peripheral erythema, due to inflammation and erythrocyte extravasation, appear as pinkish homogeneous areas. Finally, hemorrhagic crusts correspond to occasional bleeding by trauma.[1,6] Three main dermatoscopic patterns of angiokeratomas have been described: pattern 1, the most frequently observed, consists of dark lacunae and whitish veil; pattern 2 shows dark lacunae, whitish veil, and peripheral erythema; pattern 3 includes dark lacunae, whitish veil, and hemorrhagic crusts.[1]

Dermatoscopy may be useful for the differential diagnosis of angiokeratoma with a variety of skin tumors that may appear clinically similar, such as melanocytic nevi, Spitz-Reed nevi, malignant melanomas, pigmented basal cell

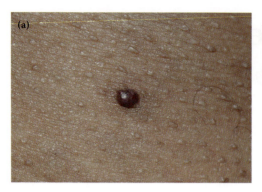
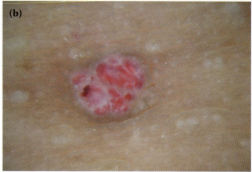

FIGURE 23.1 Solitary angiokeratoma. (a) Clinical aspect. (b) Dermatoscopy showing red lacunae and whitish veil (×10).

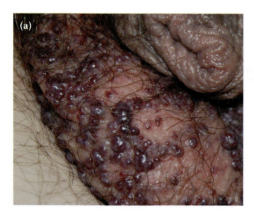
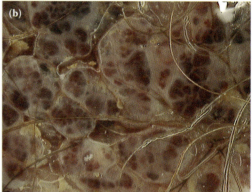

FIGURE 23.2 Angiokeratomas of the scrotum. (a) Clinical aspect. (b) Dermatoscopy showing red lacunae and whitish veil (×20).

carcinomas, seborrheic keratoses, dermatofibromas, and other vascular lesions including hemangiomas and pyogenic granulomas.

REFERENCES

1. Zaballos P, Daufì C, Puig S, et al. Dermoscopy of solitary angiokeratomas: A morphological study. *Arch Dermatol.* 2007;143:318–25.
2. Mittal R, Aggarwa A, Srivastava G. Angiokeratoma circumscriptum: A case report and review of the literature. *Int J Dermatol.* 2005;44:1031–34.
3. Zampetti A, Orteu CH, Antuzzi D, et al. Angiokeratoma: Decision-making aid for the diagnosis of Fabry disease. *Br J Dermatol.* 2012;166:712–20.
4. Wolf IH. Dermoscopic diagnosis of vascular lesions. *Clin Dermatol.* 2002;20:273–75.
5. Kim JH, Kim MR, Lee SH, et al. Dermoscopy: A useful tool for the diagnosis of angiokeratoma. *Ann Dermatol.* 2012;24:468–71.
6. Micali G, Lacarrubba F. Augmented diagnostic capability using videodermatoscopy on selected infectious and non-infectious penile growths. *Int J Dermatol.* 2011;50:1501–5.

24 Nonpigmented skin lesions
Sebaceous hyperplasia

Pedro Zaballos Diego

DEFINITION

Sebaceous hyperplasia (SH) is the most common proliferative abnormality of the sebaceous glands.

EPIDEMIOLOGY/ETIOPATHOGENESIS

SHs begin to appear in the fifth or sixth decade of a person's life and continue to appear into later life. However, premature or familial cases have been reported in which younger individuals are affected with multiple lesions, suggesting a genetic predisposition. SH incidence significantly increases in transplant patients, particularly males following heart and renal transplantation, and this may be related to immunosuppressive therapy. It has been reported in association with internal malignancy in the setting of Muir-Torre syndrome. SH has no direct association with malignant degeneration and is not a cause of morbidity; therefore, it is often found incidentally upon examination.

CLINICAL PRESENTATION/DIAGNOSIS

Classically, SH appears as a whitish-yellow or skin-colored, soft papule that may vary in size from 2–10 mm. It may be umbilicated. Rarely reported variants include a giant form, a linear or zosteriform arrangement, a diffuse form, and a familial form. Lesions may occur individually, in groups, or as a sheet of papules. Juxtaclavicular beaded lines are an additional variant characterized by closely placed papules arranged in parallel rows. SH most often presents on the face of older adults, particularly males. The forehead and cheeks are predominantly affected, and occasionally diffuse facial involvement occurs. Other less common sites include the mouth, nose, upper arms, chest, areola, penis, and vulva.

Clinically, the primary entities that must be included in the differential diagnosis of SH are basal cell carcinoma, fibrous papule of the face, milia, molluscum contagiosum, and other adnexal tumors,[1–2] and dermatoscopy may be useful as a noninvasive tool to distinguish between them, reducing unnecessary surgery.

DERMATOSCOPY/VIDEODERMATOSCOPY FEATURES

At dermatoscopy, SH shows a pattern composed of the presence of aggregated white-yellowish globules in the center of the lesions with a surrounding crown of vessels (Figures 24.1–24.7).[3–7] The central aggregated white-yellowish structures or globules, showing a sharp difference from surrounding skin, were defined by Bryden and colleagues[3] as the "cumulus sign," a descriptive sign, because these structures resemble the cumulus clouds. They histopathologically correspond to hyperplastic sebaceous glands. Bryden and colleagues[3] and Oztas and colleagues[5] observed these structures in 100% of SHs. These aggregated yellowish globules are not limited solely to SH and may also be seen in some molluscum contagiosum, nevus sebaceous of Jadassohn, and sebaceous adenoma.[7–9] Sometimes, the ostium of the gland is visible as a small crater or umbilication in the center of these yellowish structures. Oztas and colleagues[5] named the association of the central umbilication surrounded by cumulus sign as "bonbon toffee sign" and found this pattern in 80% of SHs (Figures 24.4 and 24.5). With regard to the vascular structures that can be found at the periphery of SHs, the most common ones are the "crown vessels" (Figures 24.1–24.6).[3–7] These vascular structures have been defined as

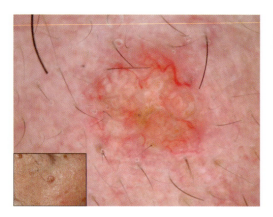

FIGURE 24.1 Dermatoscopy of sebaceous hyperplasia: aggregated white-yellowish globules in the center of the lesion ("cumulus sign") with surrounding crown of vessels; brownish globular structures with ring-like appearance in the center of the lesion can also be observed (×10).

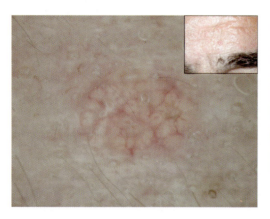

FIGURE 24.2 Typical dermatoscopic features of sebaceous hyperplasia (×10).

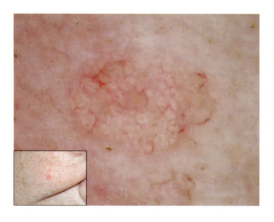

FIGURE 24.3 Typical dermatoscopic features of sebaceous hyperplasia (×10).

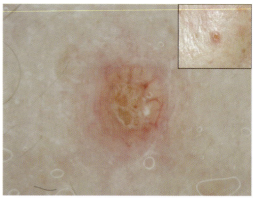

FIGURE 24.4 Dermatoscopy of sebaceous hyperplasia: the "bonbon toffee sign." A peripheral crown of vessels, characteristic of this tumor, can be observed (×10).

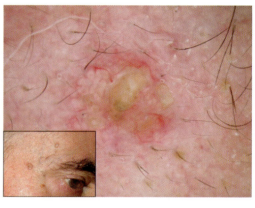

FIGURE 24.5 Dermatoscopy of sebaceous hyperplasia: the "bonbon toffee sign" and a peripheral crown of vessels (×10).

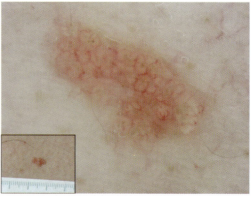

FIGURE 24.6 Dermatoscopy of large sebaceous hyperplasia: presence of aggregated white-yellowish globules and groups of orderly, bending, scarcely branching vessels located throughout the lesion (×10).

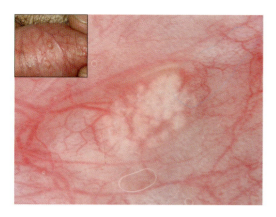

FIGURE 24.7 Typical dermatoscopic features of sebaceous hyperplasia located on the penis (×10).

groups of orderly, bending, scarcely branching vessels located along the border of the lesion.[10] These vessels may extend toward the center but do not usually cross it. They are very common in SHs, although they may be present in some cases of molluscum contagiosum. Argenziano and colleagues[10] and Oztas and colleagues[5] found crown vessels in 83.3% and 86.7% of cases, respectively. Other vascular structures that can be observed are arborizing vessels in 16.7% of cases according to Argenziano's team.[10] SH is frequently clinically misdiagnosed as basal cell carcinoma, and arborizing telangiectasias are among the characteristic criteria of this tumor. However, none of the other specific criteria of basal cell carcinoma[11] (blue globules; large, blue-gray, ovoid nests; leaf-like areas; spoke-wheel structures; and ulceration) have been found in SH, and aggregated white-yellowish globules are not typical of basal cell carcinoma. Finally, brown dots and globules, some with a ring-like appearance and milia-like cysts, are less common features that can be seen in few SHs.

REFERENCES

1. Lazar AJF, McKee PH. Tumors and related lesions of the sebaceous glands. In: Calonje E, Brenner E, Lazar A, McKee PH. *McKee's Pathology of the Skin with Clinical Correlations*. China: Elsevier Mosby; 2012. p. 1488–1507.
2. Simpson NB, Cunliffe WJ. Disorders of the sebaceous glands. In: Burns T, Breathnach S, Cox N, Griffiths C, eds. *Rook's Textbook of Dermatology*. Oxford: Blackwell, 2004. pp. 43.1–43.74.
3. Bryden AM, Dawe RS, Fleming C. Dermatoscopic features of benign sebaceous proliferation. *Clin Exp Dermatol*. 2004;29:676–77.
4. Zaballos P, Ara M, Puig S, Malvehy J. Dermoscopy of sebaceous hyperplasia. *Arch Dermatol*. 2005;141:808.
5. Oztas P, Polat M, Oztas M, et al. Bonbon toffee sign: A new dermatoscopic feature for sebaceous hyperplasia. *J Eur Acad Dermatol Venereol*. 2008;22:1200–2.
6. Zalaudek I, Argenziano G, Di Stefani A, et al. Dermoscopy in general dermatology. *Dermatology*. 2006;212:7–18.
7. Kim NH, Zell DS, Kolm I, et al. The dermoscopic differential diagnosis of yellow lobularlike structures. *Arch Dermatol*. 2008;144:962.
8. Morales A, Puig S, Zaballos P, Malvehy J. Dermoscopy of Molluscum contagiosum. *Arch Dermatol*. 2005;141:1644.
9. Zaballos P, Ara M, Puig S, Malvehy J. Dermoscopy of molluscum contagiosum: a useful tool for clinical diagnosis in adulthood. *J Eur Acad Dermatol Venereol*. 2006;20:482–83.
10. Argenziano G, Zalaudek I, Corona R, et al. Vascular structures in skin tumors: A dermoscopy study. *Arch Dermatol*. 2004;140:1485–89.
11. Menzies SW, Westerhoff K, Rabinovitz H, et al. Surface microscopy of pigmented basal cell carcinoma. *Arch Dermatol*. 2000;136:1012–16.

25 Nonpigmented skin lesions
Xanthomatous lesions

Pietro Rubegni, Linda Tognetti, Filomena Mandato, and Michele Fimiani

DEFINITION

The term *xanthomatous lesions* encompasses a variety of cutaneous manifestations characterized by abnormal intracellular and dermal lipid deposition. They may be signs of different lipoprotein disorders (e.g., familial or secondary dyslipidaemias) or arise without an underlying metabolic disease.

EPIDEMIOLOGY/ETIOPATHOGENESIS

Xanthomatous lesions are relatively common, but diffuse forms occur less frequently. Despite the large number of people who suffer from hyperlipidemia, only a minority will develop these lesions. They result from the permeation of circulating plasma lipoproteins through dermal capillary blood vessels followed by phagocytosis of the lipoproteins by macrophages, forming lipid-laden cells known as foam cells.

CLINICAL PRESENTATION/DIAGNOSIS

Xanthomatous lesions manifest as typically yellowish, sometimes tending to orange or blue, macules (flat xanthomas), papules (eruptive xanthomas), nodules (tuberous xanthomas), or tendon infiltrations (tendon xanthomas).[1] Their histology is characterized by accumulation of xanthomatous cells (macrophages) containing lipids responsible for their color. Sometimes they are idiopathic, but they are more commonly encountered in patients with internal diseases, especially in those with high cardiovascular risk.[2] Since xanthomatous lesions often indicate the concomitance of secondary or acquired hyperlipidemia, these patients should undergo a lipid profile analysis. In rare cases, they may be part of a complex syndrome (Table 25.1).[3–6]

Xanthelasms are the most frequent xanthomatous lesions. They present as yellowish papules, usually arranged symmetrically at the internal canthus of the eye, on the upper eyelids, and sometimes on the lower ones. If untreated, they may join up to form plaques that need to be removed to avoid ectropion.[7–8] In about 50% of cases, xanthelasms are an indication of hyperlipoproteinemia, usually hereditary hypercholesterolemia or dysbetalipoproteinemia. *Tuberous xanthomas* are hard, yellowish, slowly evolving nodules, often surrounded by an erythematous halo. They are generally located symmetrically in pressure regions (elbows, knees, and ankles) and are always associated with genetic (hereditary dysbetalipoproteinemia or hypercholesterolemia), secondary (cirrhosis, diabetes, endocrine disorders, obesity, nephrotic syndrome), or iatrogenic (therapy with retinoids or estrogens) hyperlipoproteinemia. *Eruptive papular xanthomas* are small inflammatory-like papules that erupt on the elbows or knees and are sometimes itchy. Initially red, the papules veer to yellowish and may unite to form tuberous/eruptive xanthomas.[9] They are usually an indication of untreated diabetes, hyperestrogenism, or alcoholism accompanied by high blood triglycerides, and may be associated with a variety of genetic hyperlipoproteinemia. *Diffuse flat normolipidemic xanthomas* are large yellowish papular plaques with well-defined borders that occur on the face, trunk, neck, elbows, and folds (Figure 25.1a). They are not associated with dyslipidemia and may be idiopathic. However, in most cases they are associated with blood disorders (especially multiple myeloma, chronic myelomonocytic leukemia, and Sezary

TABLE 25.1
Syndromes associated with skin xanthomas

Syndrome	Clinical symptoms and signs
Necrobiotic xanthoma	Purplish inflammatory plaques and nodules with a xanthomatous central area (chest and periorbital) associated with paraproteinemia in 80% of cases; they may be associated with other hematological disorders but not dyslipidemia
Montgomery disseminated xanthoma	Papular xanthomas of the skin (neck, folds, periorbital and perioral) and mucosa (pharynx, larynx) associated with diabetes insipidus in 30% of cases
Cerebrotendinous xanthomatosis	Rare autosomal dominant hereditary disease characterized by xanthelasmas, tendon xanthomas, and tuberous xanthomas. Young patients also have mental retardation, progressive spasticity, cataracts, and high cardiovascular risk. The disorder is caused by diffuse deposition of cholesterol and cholestanol.

syndrome), atopic dermatitis or Fordyce angiokeratoma.[10–11]

Juvenile xanthogranuloma is the most frequent non-Langerhans histiocytosis and consists of hard, yellow to orange papules or nodules with clear borders, usually on the face or neck (Figure 25.2a).[12–14] It is more frequent in children, although it may be also observed in adults. It may be isolated or eruptive, and micro (0.2–0.5 cm) or macro (1–3 cm) nodular. The micronodular eruptive form (60% of cases) is occasionally

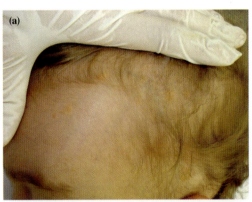

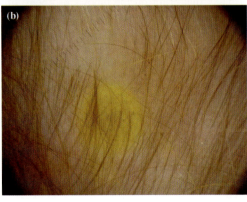

FIGURE 25.1 (a) Diffuse flat normolipidemic xanthomas. (b) Dermatoscopic examination showing pale yellow deposits.

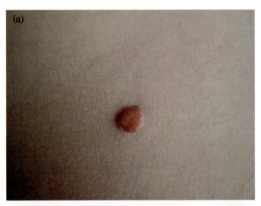

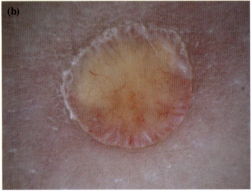

FIGURE 25.2 (a) Juvenile xanthogranuloma. (b) Dermatoscopy showing an orange-yellow background with "clouds" of paler yellow deposits; branched and linear vessels running from the periphery to the centre of the lesions are also visible.

Nonpigmented Skin Lesions

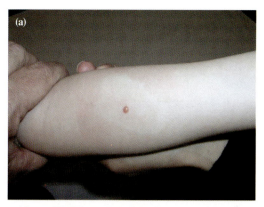

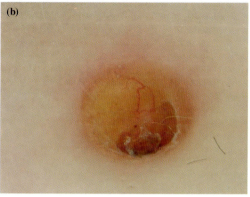

FIGURE 25.3 (a) Solitary rethiculohistiocytoma. (b) Dermatoscopy revealing branched and linear vessels predominantly at the periphery of the lesion on an orange-yellow background.

associated with eye involvement, neurofibromatosis, or juvenile chronic myeloid leukemia, whereas the macronodular form may indicate liver or kidney distress. Xanthogranulomas are not associated with dyslipidemias, unlike many other xanthomatous lesions.

Reticulohistiocytoma, also known as solitary epithelioid histiocytoma, is a localized benign form of histiocytosis that generally occurs in young adults or middle-aged people. It presents as an asymptomatic, reddish, dermal nodule that may spontaneously resolve over a period of months to years (Figure 25.3a).

Finally, the term *xanthomization* indicates a gradual process of accumulation of lipids in tumoral lesions such as histiocytomas or inflammatory sequelae such as lipid necrobiosis, foreign body reaction, histiocytosis X, erythema elevatum diutinum, and leprosy scars.

DERMATOSCOPY/ VIDEODERMATOSCOPY FEATURES

Generally, xanthomatous lesions show similar patterns by dermatoscope.[15] Typical findings include a yellowish background that may vary from pale yellow to orange (Figures 25.1b, 25.2b, 25.3b, and 25.4), and vessels (linear branched, in most cases) disposed at the periphery.[15–16] During dermatoscopic examination, undue pressure of the dermatoscope on the skin may limit blood flow to the lesion and prevent observation of the vascular component.[17–18] Apart from these two features, xanthomas have no other specific dermatoscopic characteristics, though some lesions may show other details.

Juvenile xanthogranuloma is characterized by a homogeneous background with various shades of yellow and orange (*sign of the setting sun*, expression of the presence of xanthomatous histiocytes).[15] Palmer and colleagues also described "clouds" of pale yellow deposits.[16] When minimal pressure is exerted on the dermatoscope, branched linear[17] or isolated dotted vessels,[15] running from the periphery to the center of the lesions, can be observed (Figure 25.2b).

Reticulohistiocytoma usually shows a yellowish background, or a uniformly yellow central area and a pink-orange color in the periphery. Light-brown globules[15] or "clouds of paler yellow deposits"[18] can be present, along with branched[18] vessels located at the periphery of the lesion (Figure 25.4). Brownish globules correspond to dots of hemosiderin in the upper dermis.[15] In many cases, reticulohistiocytoma shows aspects

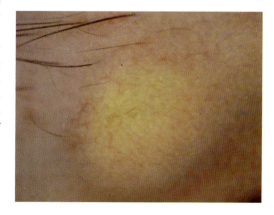

FIGURE 25.4 Dermatoscopy of xanthelasms revealing only a yellow background.

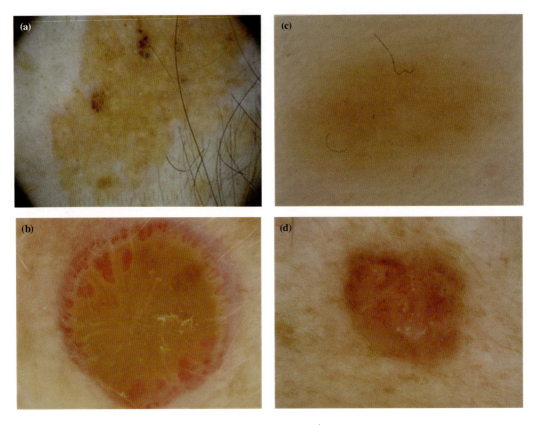

FIGURE 25.5 Dermatoscopy of sebaceous nevus (a), Spitz nevus (b), Bowen's disease (c), and basal cell carcinoma (d). All these lesions reveal yellowish structures that resemble those observed in xanthomatous lesions.

similar to the juvenile xanthogranuloma, such as the sign of the setting sun;[19] hence the differential diagnosis is usually difficult. Notably, three different reticulohistiocytoma patterns (brown reticular structures, central white scar-like patches, and the "setting-sun" pattern) were described in the same patient with multicentric reticulohistiocytosis.[20] In addition, a new dermatoscopic feature, characterized by central white-grayish area and white-pinkish streaks situated at the periphery, without dilated vessels, has been reported by de Oliveira and colleagues.[21]

Xanthomized dermatofibroma often reveal, along with the omogeneous yellow pattern due to dermal xanthomatous deposits, a peripheral delicate pigment network (which is usually seen in typical dermatofibromas), corresponding to hyperplastic epidermis with basal hyperpigmentation.[15,22]

Xanthomatous lesions should be differentiated from a number of cutaneous neoformations that sometimes show a yellowish background, or yellow structures, when observed under the dermatoscope. Sebaceous hyperplasia is usually characterized by yellow lobular-like structures or aggregated yellow globules.[23] However, these features are not specific, as they can be observed in nevus sebaceous of Jadassohn (Figure 25.5a) and sebaceous adenoma (Muir-Torre syndrome) as well. In those cases, yellow lobules correspond to dermal conglomerations of sebaceous glands. Spitz nevus can show a diffuse yellowish pigmented network (Figure 25.5b), while balloon cell nevus, as reported by Cinotti and colleagues, may present yellow globules and overlapping structureless brown areas.[24] Bowen's disease lesion also can reveal a yellowish opaque surface due to relevant keratinization (Figure 25.5c).[25] A considerable number of basal cell carcinomas demonstrate yellowish structures, including milia-like cystis and yellow globules (8% and 42%, respectively, of the case study analyzed by Bellucci et al.).[26] Finally, describing the dermatoscopic morphology of apocrine hidrocystomas, Zaballos and colleagues assessed the presence of a yellow homogeneous central area in 32% of cases.[27]

REFERENCES

1. De Schaetzen V, Richert B, De La Brassinne M. Les xanthomes. *Rev Med Liege.* 2004;59:46–50.
2. Crook M. Xanthelasma and cardiovascular risk. *Int J Clin Pract.* 2008;62:178–79.
3. Fernández-Herrera J, Pedraz J. Necrobiotic xanthogranuloma. *Semin Cutan Med Surg.* 2007;26:108–13.
4. Shah KC, Poonnoose SI, George R, et al. Necrobiotic xanthogranuloma with cutaneous and cerebral manifestations. Case report and review of the literature. *J Neurosurg.* 2004;100:1111–14.
5. Kumakiri M, Sudoh M, Miura Y. Xanthoma disseminatum. Report of a case, with histological and ultrastructural studies of skin lesions. *J Am Acad Dermatol.* 1981;4:291–99.
6. Romero JO, Callejón JR, Alonso G. Cerebrotendinous xanthomatosis. *Neurologia.* 2008;23:530–31.
7. Rohrich RJ, Janis JE, Pownell PH. Xanthelasma palpebrarum: A review and current management principles. *Plast Reconstr Surg.* 2002;110:1310–14.
8. Singla A. Normolipemic papular xanthoma with xanthelasma. *Dermatol Online. J* 2006;12:19.
9. Merola JF, Mengden SJ, Soldano A, Rosenman K. Eruptive xanthomas. *Dermatol Online. J* 2008;14:10.
10. Breier F, Zelger B, Reiter H, et al. Papular xanthoma: A clinicopathological study of 10 cases. *J Cutan Pathol.* 2002;29:200–6.
11. Caputo R, Passoni E, Cavicchini S. Papular xanthoma associated with angiokeratoma of Fordyce: Considerations on the nosography of this rare non-Langerhans cell histiocytoxanthomatosis. *Dermatology.* 2003;206:165–68.
12. Shoo BA, Shinkai K, McCalmont TH, Fox LP. Xanthogranulomas associated with hematologic malignancy in adulthood. *J Am Acad Dermatol.* 2008;59:488–93.
13. Satter EK, Gendernalik SB, Galeckas KJ. Diffuse xanthogranulomatous dermatitis and systemic Langerhans cell histiocytosis: A novel case that demonstrates bridging between the non-Langerhans cell histiocytosis and Langerhans cell histiocytosis. *J Am Acad Dermatol.* 2009;60:841–48.
14. Navajas B, Eguino P, Trébol I, et al. Multiple adult xanthogranuloma. *Actas Dermosifiliogr.* 2005;96:171–74.
15. Cavicchini S, Tourlaki A, Tanzi C, Alessi E. Dermoscopy of solitary yellow lesions in adults. *Arch Dermatol.* 2008;144:1412.
16. Palmer A, Bowling J. Dermoscopic appearance of juvenile xanthogranuloma. *Dermatology.* 2007;215:256-9.
17. Rubegni P, Mandato F, Fimiani M. Juvenile xanthogranuloma: Dermoscopic pattern. *Dermatology.* 2009;218:380.
18. Rubegni P, Mandato F, Mourmouras V, et al. Xanthomatous papule in a child. Solitary reticulohistiocytoma (SRH). *Clin Exp Dermatol.* 2010;35:e58–59.
19. Hussain SH, Kozic H, JB Lee. The utility of dermatoscopy in the evaluation of xanthogranulomas. *Pediatr Dermatol.* 2008;25:505–6.
20. Kaçar N, Tasli L, Argenziano G, Demirkan N. Reticulohistiocytosis: Different dermatoscopic faces and a good response to methotrexate treatment. *Clin Exper Dermatol.* 2010;35:e120–22.
21. De Oliveira FL, Nogueira LL, Chaves GM, et al. A unique dermoscopy pattern of solitary cutaneous reticulohistiocytosis. *Case Rep Dermatol Med.* 2013;2013:674896.
22. Zaballos P, Puig S, Llambrich A, Malvehy J. Dermoscopy of dermatofibromas: A prospective morphological study of 412 cases. *Arch Dermatol.* 2008;144:75–83.
23. Kim NH, Zell DS, Kolm I, et al. The dermoscopic differential diagnosis of yellow lobular-like structures. *Arch Dermatol.* 2008;144:962.
24. Cinotti E, Perrot JL, Labeille B, et al. Yellow globules in balloon cell naevus. *Australasian J Dermatol.* 2013;54:268–70.
25. Fargnoli MC, Kostaki D, Piccioni A, et al. Dermoscopy in the diagnosis and management of non-melanoma skin cancers. *Eur J Dermatol.* 2012;22:456–63.
26. Bellucci C, Arginelli F, Bassoli S, et al. Dermoscopic yellow structures in basal cell carcinoma. *J Eur Acad Dermatol Venereol.* 2014;28:651–54.
27. Zaballos P, Bañuls J, Medina C, et al. Dermoscopy of apocrine hidrocystomas: a morphological study. *J Eur Acad Dermatol Venereol.* 2014;28:378–81.

26 Nonpigmented skin lesions
Porokeratosis

Pedro Zaballos Diego

DEFINITION

The term *porokeratosis* encompasses a variety of clonal disorders of keratinization characterized by marginate scaling lesions. Five clinical variants of porokeratosis are recognized: classic porokeratosis of Mibelli, disseminated superficial actinic porokeratosis (DSAP), porokeratosis palmaris et plantaris disseminata, linear porokeratosis, and punctate porokeratosis.[1–3]

EPIDEMIOLOGY/ETIOPATHOGENESIS

Porokeratoses are genetically heterogeneous disorders with several loci identified; however, most cases appear to be sporadic. The pathogenetic mechanisms still remain unknown. Several risk factors for the development of porokeratosis have been identified, including ultraviolet radiation and immunosuppression.

CLINICAL PRESENTATION/DIAGNOSIS

Porokeratosis is clinically characterized by sharply demarcated, atrophic, annular lesions with a distinct keratotic edge corresponding histologically to the presence of the cornoid lamella, a thin column of tightly packed parakeratotic cells within a keratin-filled epidermal invagination.

DSAP is the most common presentation, with many lesions of up to 10 mm, predominantly in sun-exposed sites in middle-aged individuals in their third or fourth decade of life, especially those with sun-sensitive skin. DSAP is three times more likely to develop in women than in men. The tendency to develop these lesions is inherited as an autosomical dominant trait. Multiple, annular, keratotic lesions that develop predominantly on the extensor surfaces of the legs and the arms characterize DSAP. The lesion begins as a 1- to 3-mm conical papule, reddish or brownish in color, that contains a keratotic plug that expands to a sharp, slightly raised, keratotic ring, producing a plaque of 10 mm or more. The skin within the ring is usually somewhat atrophic and mildly reddened or hyperpigmented. In a few cases, the center of the area becomes inflamed, covered by thick hyperkeratosis, or even ulcerated and crusted. The lesions are usually asymptomatic but may itch slightly. There is a nonactinic form of disseminated, superficial porokeratosis after organ transplantation, renal failure, HIV infection, or in association with other causes of immunosuppression that may have a generalized distribution of identical lesions, sparing the palms and the soles.[1–3]

The formation of squamous or basal cell carcinomas has been reported in all forms of porokeratosis, although the degree of premalignant potential is controversial.

DERMATOSCOPY/VIDEODERMATOSCOPY FEATURES

Dermatoscopy of porokeratosis reveals a whitish annular structure called a "white track" located at the periphery of the lesion, with a brownish pigmentation on the inner side and with a double white track in some areas (Figures 26.1–26.7).[4–7] The color of this annular structure could be yellowish or light brown in rare cases. This single or double white track is characteristic of porokeratosis and corresponds histopathologically to the cornoid lamella. The papillary dermis beneath the cornoid lamella contains a moderately dense, lymphocytic infiltrate and dilated capillaries. Therefore, brownish pigmentation on the inner side of the white track and a peripheral vascularization may be

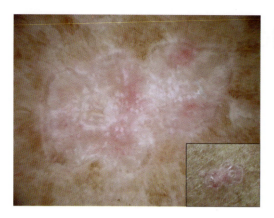

FIGURE 26.1 Dermatoscopy of porokeratosis: peripheral white track that demarcates a central, red-whitish, homogeneous area with dotted vessels and scales (×10).

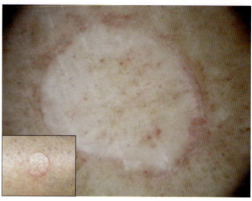

FIGURE 26.3 Dermatoscopy of porokeratosis: peripheral white track and a central, whitish, homogeneous area, with dotted vessels, red globules and a delicate pigment network (×10).

observed. Liquefactive degeneration of the basal layer of the epithelium is sometimes present and occasionally provokes melanophagia, and, in these cases, some blue-gray coarse granules can be observed.

The white track demarcates a central, light-whitish, homogeneous area with different kinds of vessels (red dots and globules, linear-irregular vessels, or telangiectasias) (Figures 26.1–26.5) that are more easily observed because of the presence of atrophic epithelium in the center of the porokeratosis.[4–7] The epithelium toward the center may be of normal thickness or even acanthotic; because of this, in less common cases, an intense white homogeneous area or even a verrucous surface can be observed (Figures 26.6–26.7). Other uncommon structures that can be seen in the center of the porokeratosis are a delicate pigment network or brown globules, some of them with a ring-like appearance. The lesions of DSAP may be clinically interpreted as actinic keratoses or psoriatic plaques. Four essential dermatoscopic features can be observed in nonpigmented actinic keratosis that combine to produce the "strawberry" pattern: erythema, revealing a marked, pink-to-red "pseudo network" surrounding the hair follicles; white-to-yellow surface scale; fine, linear-wavy vessels surrounding the hair follicles; and hair

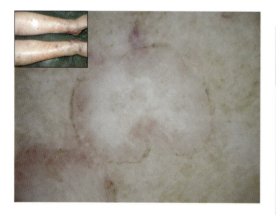

FIGURE 26.2 Dermatoscopy of porokeratosis: peripheral white-brownish track and a central, whitish, homogeneous area; in some areas peripheral vascular structures can also be observed (×10).

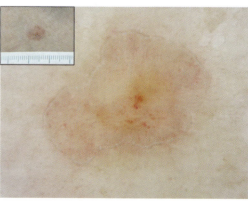

FIGURE 26.4 Dermatoscopy of porokeratosis: white track and a central area with dotted vessels and red globules (×10).

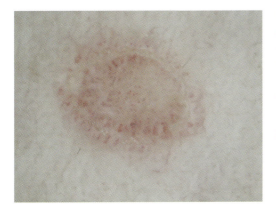

FIGURE 26.5 Dermatoscopy of porokeratosis: peripheral white track with different kinds of vessels (×10).

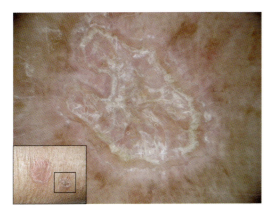

FIGURE 26.6 Dermatoscopy of porokeratosis: peripheral white track with a central scaly surface (×10).

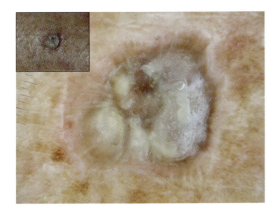

FIGURE 26.7 Dermatoscopy of porokeratosis: verrucous surface in the center of the lesion, corresponding to acanthotic epidermis (×10).

follicle openings filled with yellowish keratotic plugs and/or surrounded by a white halo.[8-9] The dermatoscopic pattern associated with psoriasis is composed of multiple, uniformly sized and distributed dotted vessels or red globules, together with a central surface scale.[10-11]

REFERENCES

1. Judge MR, Malean WHI, Munro CS. Disorders of keratinization. In: Burns T, Breathnach S, Cox N, Griffiths C, eds. *Rook´s Textbook of Dermatology*. Oxford: Blackwell; 2004. pp. 34.75–7.
2. Shumack SP, Commens CA. Disseminated superficial actinic porokeratosis: A clinical study. *J Am Acad Dermatol*. 1989;20:1015–22.
3. Sasson M, Krain AD. Porokeratosis and cutaneous malignancy. A review. *Dermatol Surg*. 1996;22:339–42.
4. Delfino M, Argenziano G, Nino M. Dermoscopy for the diagnosis of porokeratosis. *J Eur Acad Dermatol Venereol*. 2004;18:194–95.
5. Zaballos P, Puig S, Malvehy J. Dermoscopy of disseminated superficial actinic porokeratosis. *Arch Dermatol*. 2004;140(11):1410.
6. Panasiti V, Rossi M, Curzio M, et al. Disseminated superficial actinic porokeratosis diagnosed by dermoscopy. *Int J Dermatol*. 2008;47:308–10.
7. Vargas-Laguna E, Nagore E, Alfaro A, et al. Monitoring the evolution of a localized type of porokeratosis using dermatoscopy. *Actas Dermosifiliogr*. 2006;97:77–78.
8. Zalaudek I, Giacomel J, Argenziano G, et al. Dermoscopy of facial nonpigmented actinic keratosis. *Br J Dermatol*. 2006;155:951–56.
9. Peris K, Micantonio T, Piccolo D, Fargnoli MC. Dermoscopic features of actinic keratosis. *J Dtsch Dermatol Ges*. 2007;5:970–76.
10. Vázquez-López F, Manjón-Haces JA, Maldonado-Seral C, et al. Dermoscopic features of plaque psoriasis and lichen planus: new observations. *Dermatology*. 2003;207:151–56.
11. Zalaudek I, Argenziano G, Di Stefani A, et al. Dermoscopy in general dermatology. *Dermatology*. 2006;212:7–18.

27 Nonpigmented skin lesions
Apocrine hidrocystoma

Pedro Zaballos Diego

DEFINITION

Apocrine hidrocystoma (AH) is a benign, cystic proliferation of the apocrine secretory glands.

EPIDEMIOLOGY/ETIOPATHOGENESIS

AH is uncommon, showing an equal sex incidence and arising most often in the middle aged. The pathogenesis is unknown. Possible causes include occlusion or blockage of the sweat ducts.

CLINICAL PRESENTATION/DIAGNOSIS

AH presents as an asymptomatic, intradermal, dome-shaped, translucent nodule with a smooth surface (Figures 27.1–27.2), and its color ranges from flesh-colored to blue-black ("hidrocystoma noir").[1] It is usually found on the head and neck, commonly affecting the periorbital area or cheeks. AH is most often solitary, but multiple lesions have also been documented sporadically or associated with the Schöpf-Schulz-Passarge syndrome, in which small lesions typically involve the margins of both eyelids. The clinical diagnosis of AH is usually straightforward. However, because of its color, it may mimic pigmented basal cell carcinoma or melanocytic lesions, including melanoma.[2] Histologically, AH is a large unilocular or multilocular dermal cystic space, usually without connection to the overlying epidermis, typically lined by a double layer of epithelial cells, with the outer layer consisting of myoepithelial cells and inner layer consisting of tall columnar cells. "Decapitation" secretion, which is typical of apocrine glands, is usually present.[1]

DERMATOSCOPY/VIDEODERMATOSCOPY FEATURES

Dermatoscopy may be useful for the diagnosis of AH (Figures 27.3–27.7). A study revealed that the association of a homogeneous area that occupies the whole lesion with arborizing vessels is the most common dermatoscopic pattern associated with AH, as it was identified in 15 of 22 lesions (68.2% of cases).[3] Other specific criteria for melanocytic or nonmelanocytic tumors were absent.

The dermatoscopic color of the homogeneous area, which histopathologically corresponds to the large unilocular or multilocular cystic space situated within the dermis, varies from skin-colored (31.8% of cases) to pink (4.5%), yellow (31.8%), gray (4.5%), or blue (22.7%).[3] The cause of the blue coloration, which may be observed in clinically pigmented AH, is unknown. Some authors have related it to the presence of lipofuscin, melanin, or iron in the cysts; others suggest the hypothesis of the Tyndall phenomenon, as pigmented AH is generally associated with larger or multilocular cystic spaces.[4] Bluish homogeneous pigmentation of the whole lesion can also be observed at dermatoscopy in blue nevus, nodular or metastatic melanoma, aneurismal dermatofibroma, trichilemmal cyst, basal cell carcinoma, and rarely in some Spitz/Reed nevi.[5]

Arborizing vessels represent the most common vascular structures observed in AH (68.2%) followed by linear-irregular vessels (9.1%).[3] Arborizing vessels are defined as "in focus" telangiectasias with distinct tree-like ramifications and are generally associated with basal

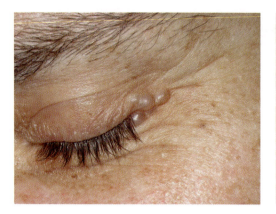

FIGURE 27.1 Apocrine hidrocystoma of the left periorbital area in a 48-year-old man.

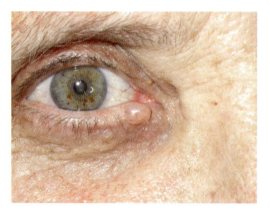

FIGURE 27.2 Apocrine hidrocystoma of the right lower eyelid in a 65-year-old man.

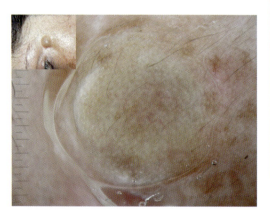

FIGURE 27.3 Dermatoscopy of apocrine hidrocystoma: yellowish homogeneous area that occupies the entire lesion and small arborizing vessels (×10).

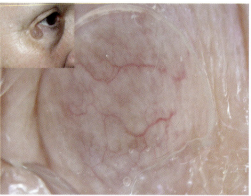

FIGURE 27.4 Dermatoscopy of apocrine hidrocystoma: skin-colored homogeneous area that occupies the entire lesion and arborizing telangiectasias, which are indistinguishable from those found in basal cell carcinomas (×10).

cell carcinoma,[6–7] although they also may be observed in other lesions, such as dermal nevi, sebaceous hyperplasias, pigmented poromas, xanthogranulomas, and leishmaniasis.[8]

Finally, chrysalis or shiny white streaks are found in 22.7% of AH.[3] These white, linear structures only visible with polarized dermatoscopy may be observed in melanomas, Spitz/Reed nevi, dermatofibromas, and basal cell carcinomas,[9] and their histological substrate is believed to be dermal fibrosis. Changes in the

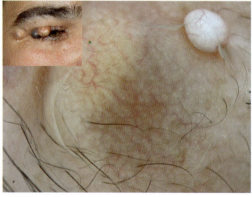

FIGURE 27.5 Dermatoscopy of two lesions in a 55-year-old man with multiple apocrine hidrocystomas of the eyelids: the homogeneous area is yellowish in the big one and white in the small one. Both of them have arborizing telangiectasias (×10).

Nonpigmented Skin Lesions

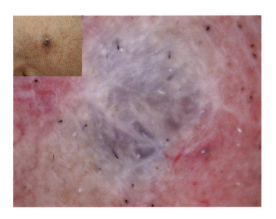

FIGURE 27.6 Dermatoscopy of pigmented apocrine hidrocystoma ("hidrocystoma noir"): bluish homogeneous area that occupies the entire lesion and presence of chrysalis (×10).

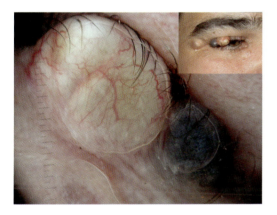

FIGURE 27.7 Dermatoscopy of other two apocrine hidrocystomas of patient seen in Figure 27.5.

orientation of collagen fibers due to the pressure of the large dermal cysts could be an explanation of this phenomenon.[3]

REFERENCES

1. Brenn T, McKee PH. Tumors of the sweat glands. In: Calonje E, Brenner E, Lazar A, McKee PH, eds. *McKee's Pathology of the Skin with Clinical Correlations.* China: Elsevier Mosby; 2012. pp. 1508-70.
2. Anzai S, Goto M, Fujiwara S, Da T. Apocrine hidrocystoma: A case report and analysis of 167 Japanese cases. *Int J Dermatol.* 2005;44:702–3.
3. Zaballos P, Bañuls J, Medina C, et al. Dermoscopy of apocrine hidrocystomas: A morphological study. *J Eur Acad Dermatol Venereol.* 2014;28:378–81.
4. Malhotra R, Bhawan J. The nature of pigment in pigmented apocrine hidrocystoma. *J Cutan Pathol.* 1985;12:106–9.
5. Scope A, Benvenuto-Andrade C, et al. Nonmelanocytic lesions defying the two-step dermoscopy algorithm. *Dermatol Surg.* 2006 32:1398–406.
6. Menzies SW, Westerhoff K, Rabinovitz H, et al. Surface microscopy of pigmented basal cell carcinoma. *Arch Dermatol.* 2000;136:1012–16.
7. Altamura D, Menzies SW, Argenziano G, et al. Dermatoscopy of basal cell carcinoma: Morphologic variability of global and local features and accuracy of diagnosis. *J Am Acad Dermatol.* 2010;62:67–75.
8. Zalaudek I, Kreusch J, Giacomel J, et al. How to diagnose nonpigmented skin tumors: A review of vascular structures seen with dermoscopy: Part II. Nonmelanocytic skin tumors. *J Am Acad Dermatol.* 2010;63:377–86.
9. Marghoob AA, Cowell L, Kopf AW, Scope A. Observation of chrysalis structures with polarized dermoscopy. *Arch Dermatol.* 2009;145:618.

28 Nonpigmented skin lesions
Bowen's disease

Leonardo Bugatti and Giorgio Filosa

DEFINITION

Bowen's disease (BD) is an intraepidermal (*in situ*) squamous cell carcinoma.

EPIDEMIOLOGY/ETIOPATHOGENESIS

BD predominantly affects older female patients, and in about three-quarters of the cases it is located on the lower limbs. Reported relevant etiological factors are irradiation (solar, photochemotherapy, radiotherapy), long-term arsenic exposure, and immunosuppression.

CLINICAL PRESENTATION/DIAGNOSIS

BD clinically presents as a slowly enlarging, sharply demarcated erythematous plaque with a crusting and scaling surface (Figure 28.1). Resemblance to psoriasis or dermatitis leads to a delay in the correct diagnosis. Lesions are usually solitary but may be multiple in 10%–20% of patients. Unusual sites or variants include subungual/periungual, palmar, genital, perineal, pigmented, and verrucous BD. Most studies suggest a risk of progression to invasive squamous cell carcinoma of about 3%–20% for classic BD.[1] Development of ulceration is usually a sign of invasive carcinoma. Histopathologically, BD is characterized by acanthotic epidermis and elongation and thickening of rete ridges, with convoluted and dilated papillary vessels. Throughout the epidermis the cells lie in complete disorder resulting in a "windblown appearance." Many cells are highly atypical, showing large hyperchromatic nuclei with conspicuous nucleoli and abundant cytoplasm. Another common feature is the presence of occasional individually atypical keratinized cells (Figure 28.2). The border between epidermis and dermis appears sharp and the basement membrane remains intact. The upper dermis shows a moderate amount of chronic inflammatory infiltrate, which sometimes adopts a lichenoid distribution.

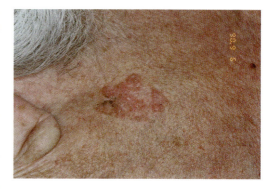

FIGURE 28.1 Bowen's disease: sharply demarcated erythemato-desquamative plaque.

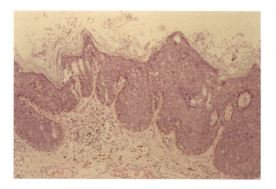

FIGURE 28.2 Histopathology picture of Bowen's disease showing epidermal acanthosis with a number of highly atypical keratinocytes often with features of dyskeratosis (H&E, ×100).

DERMATOSCOPY/ VIDEODERMATOSCOPY FEATURES

Several dermatoscopic features of BD have been described (Table 28.1). The most characteristic and common findings are represented by a multicomponent global pattern (90%–100%), atypical vascular structures (86.6%–100%), and scaly surface (64.2%–90%).[2–3]

The evaluation of vascular pattern by dermatoscopy, though not specific, has a diagnostic significance in skin tumors.[4–6] Kreusch has given a thorough morphological illustration of the vascular component of skin tumors, suggesting an algorithm for the diagnosis.[7] The recognition of distinctive vascular structures enhances the diagnostic range of dermatoscopy, especially when the classic pigmented structures are lacking, and guidelines have been established to assist in making the most appropriate management decision.[8,9] In BD, vascular structures mainly consist of dotted vessels (50%) irregularly distributed in clusters, although linear, arborizing, bushy, and hairpin-like vessels can be found (Figures 28.3-28.4). Dotted vessels histopathologically correlate with dilated tortuous capillaries of middle reticular dermis progressing to the top of the papillae. Higher magnification can disclose a distinctive type of vascular structures, namely "glomerular vessels," characterized by highly convoluted tortuous capillaries mimicking the glomerular apparatus of the kidney (Figure 28.5). Some authors distinguish between dotted and glomerular vessels, since the latter are usually larger in size, often looped, and regularly arranged in a patchy distribution (Figures 28.6–28.7).[3,10] Glomerular morphology

FIGURE 28.3 Dermatoscopy of Bowen's disease: brownish pseudonetwork, dotted and linear vascular structures (×10).

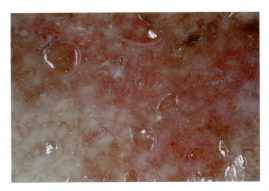

FIGURE 28.4 Dermatoscopy of Bowen's disease: dotted vascular structures, scaly surface, hemorrhages (×10).

has also been described for severe venous stasis.[11] A corona of glomerular and hairpin vessels has been described as a marker of hyperkeratotic BD (Figure 28.8).[12] It can be speculated that vascular morphology is consistent with

TABLE 28.1
Dermatoscopic features of Bowen's disease
- Multicomponent global pattern
- Atypical vascular structures (dotted/glomerular)
- Scaly surface
- Pseudonetwork
- Irregular, structureless, diffuse pigmentation
- Patchy distribution of small, brown globules
- Focal/multifocal hypopigmentation
- Blue-whitish veil
- Peppering/white areas
- Hemorrhages

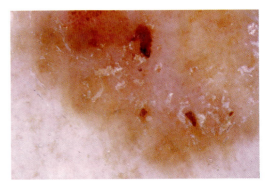

FIGURE 28.5 Dermatoscopy of Bowen's disease: multicomponent global pattern, irregular diffuse structureless pigmentation, dotted (glomerular) vascular pattern, and scaly surface (×10).

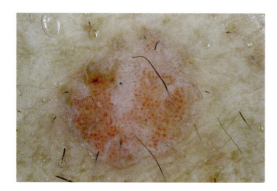

FIGURE 28.6 Dermatoscopy of Bowen's disease: dotted vascular structures and multifocal hypopigmentation (×10).

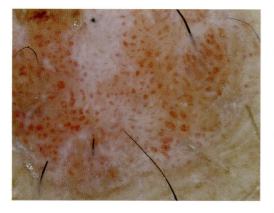

FIGURE 28.7 Dermatoscopy of Bowen's disease (magnified detail of Figure 28.6): tortuous capillaries with glomerular, hairpin, bushy morphology.

a process of tumoral neoangiogenesis in BD. Videocapillaroscopic studies might better describe the vascular structures involved in BD and other cutaneous neoplasias.

Dotted vessels can commonly be found in melanocytic tumors, sometimes in seborrheic keratoses and other skin diseases, such as psoriasis, warts, clear cell acanthoma, and dermatofibroma. In most cases of psoriasis, red dotted globules are uniformly distributed over the entire surface, whereas dotted vessels in warts are distinctive for a pale halo of keratinization.[11] Dotted vessels in clear cell acanthoma are often arranged uniformly like pearls in a line with a psoriasiform appearance.[13] In dermatofibromas, dotted vessels may be either centrally located or diffuse throughout the lesion together with other accompanying features, such as globular like-structures, a scar-like white patch, and a peripheral fine network.[14] Dotted vessels are reported to be a frequent finding in amelanotic melanoma, especially in early thin lesions. In this case the concurrence of a whitish to pinkish veil and a small amount of residual light-brown pigmentation may contribute to the diagnosis.[15–19]

The scaly surface represents another dermatoscopic finding of BD. Degree of scaling may vary according to different factors, such as body location, environmental conditions, topical pretreatment, and type of lubricant used to minimize surface reflection. The greater thickness of the corneal layer in acral skin gives rise to heavier scaling (Figure 28.9).[20]

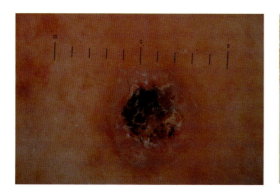

FIGURE 28.8 Dermatoscopy of a hyperkeratotic nodule of Bowen's disease: corona of glomerular vessels surrounding a central scaly plug (×10).

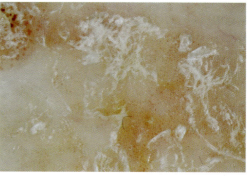

FIGURE 28.9 Dermatoscopy of Bowen's disease: dotted vascular structures, scaly surface, hemorrhages (×10).

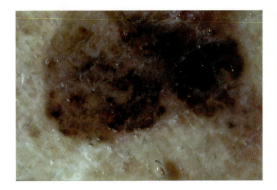

FIGURE 28.10 Dermatoscopy of pigmented Bowen's disease: scaly surface, irregular diffuse pigmentation and patchy distribution of globules (×10).

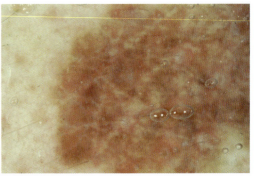

FIGURE 28.11 Dermatoscopy of pigmented Bowen's disease: pseudonetwork and irregular, structureless diffuse pigmentation (×10).

BD is generally scarcely pigmented, although pigmented structures can be detected, especially in the unusual form of heavily pigmented BD, such as the presence of pseudonetwork (10%–35.7%), irregular structureless diffuse pigmentation (64.2%–80%), and small brown globules (64.2%–90%).[2–3] The pigmented globules are usually smaller than those associated with melanocytic lesions and follow a regular patchy distribution over the lesion (Figure 28.10). A linear arrangement of brown and/or gray dots and/or coiled vessels has been described as a specific clue to pigmented BD.[21] In heavily pigmented BD, pseudo-network or reticular pigmentation, sometimes simulating atypical network or irregular flossy streaks, can be the only dermatoscopic criterion, lacking other well-expressed standard criteria (Figure 28.11).[22–23] This should trigger the prompt removal of the lesion for dermopathologic examination. The false atypical pigmented network may be created by the thickening of the rete ridges due to deposits of melanin within the tumoral cells in the dermal papillae.[24]

Dermatoscopy has also been proposed as a valuable tool for monitoring of nonsurgical treatment of BD, where the disappearance of vascular structures may indicate adequate treatment while the existence of such structures after treatment appears to be associated with persistence of the disease (Figure 28.12).[23]

In conclusion, vascular structures (dotted vessels or "glomerular" subtype morphology) and scaly surface represent valuable dermatoscopic clues to the diagnosis of BD. However, further studies are needed to assess the specificity and sensitivity of these dermatoscopic criteria in differentiating BD from other pigmented and nonpigmented skin tumors.[2–3,24]

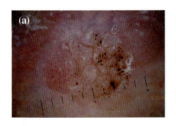
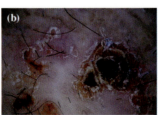
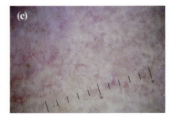

FIGURE 28.12 Dermatoscopy monitoring of Bowen's disease after photodynamic treatment; (a) time 0, (b) after one session, (c) after two sessions (×10).

REFERENCES

1. Kao GF. Carcinoma arising in Bowen's disease. *Arch Dermatol.* 1986;22:1124–26.
2. Bugatti L, Filosa G, De Angelis R. Dermoscopic observation of Bowen's disease. *J Eur Acad Dermatol Venereol.* 2004;18:572–74.
3. Zalaudek I, Argenziano G, Leinweber B, et al. Dermoscopy of Bowen's disease. *Br J Dermatol.* 2004;150;1112–16.
4. Kreusch J, Koch F. Characterization of vascular patterns in skin tumors by incident light microscopy. *Hautartz.* 1996;47:264–72.
5. Stolz W, Landthaler M, Falco OB, et al. *Color Atlas of Dermoscopy.* 2nd ed. Oxford: Blackwell Publishing, 2002.
6. Argenziano G, Fabbroncini G, Carli P, et al. Clinical and dermoscopic criteria for the preoperative evaluation of cutaneous melanoma thickness. *J Am Acad Dermatol.* 1999;40:61–68.
7. Kreusch J. Vascular patterns in skin tumors. *Clin Dermatol.* 2002;20:248–54.
8. Argenziano G, Zalaudek I, Corona R, et al. Vascular structures in skin tumors. A dermoscopy study. *Arch Dermatol.* 2004;140:1485–89.
9. Zalaudek I, Kreusch J, Giacomel J, et al. How to diagnose nonpigmented skin tumors: A review of vascular structures seen with dermoscopy. *J Am Acad Dermatol.* 2010;63.377–86.
10. Zalaudek I, Di Stefani A, Argenziano G. The specific dermoscopic criteria of Bowen's disease. *J Eur Acad Dermatol Venereol.* 2006;20:241–62.
11. Vázquez-López F, Kreush J, Marghoob AA. Dermoscopic semiology: Further insights into vascular features by screening a large spectrum of nontumoral skin lesions. *Br J Dermatol.* 2004;150:226–31.
12. Kirby W, Tarrillion M. Corona of glomerular vessels: A diagnostic marker of hyperkeratotic Bowen's disease. *Dermatol Surg.* 2013;39:1395–98.
13. Bugatti L, Filosa G, Broganelli P, Tomasini C. Psoriasis-like dermoscopic pattern of clear cell acanthoma. *J Eur Acad Dermatol Venereol.* 2003;17:452–55.
14. Zaballos P, Puig S, Llambrich A, Malvhey J. Dermoscopy of dermatofibromas: A prospective morphological study of 412 cases. *Arch Dermatol.* 2008;144:75–82.
15. Pizzichetta MA, Talamini R, Stanganelli I, et al. Amelanotic/hypomelanotic melanoma: Clinical and dermoscopic features. *Br J Dermatol.* 2004;150:1117–24.
16. Bono R, Maurichi A, Moglia D, et al. Clinical and dermatoscopic diagnosis of early amelanotic melanoma. *Melanoma Res.* 2001;491–94.
17. Zalaudek I, Argenziano G, Kerl H, et al. Amelanotic/hypomelanotic melanoma—is dermoscopy useful for diagnosis? *J Dtsch Dermatol Ges.* 2003;1:369–73.
18. Chu-Sung Hu S, Chiu H, Chen G, et al. Dermoscopy as a diagnostic and follow-up tool for pigmented Bowen's disease on acral region. *Dermatol Surg.* 2008,34:1248–53.
19. Cameron A, Rosendhal C, Tschandl P, et al. Dermatoscopy of pigmented Bowen's disease. *J Am Acad Dermatol.* 2010;62:597–604.
20. Stante M, De Giorgi V, Massi D, et al. Pigmented Bowen's disease mimicking cutaneous melanoma: Clinical and dermoscopic aspects. *Dermatol Surg.* 2004;30:541–44.
21. Takayuki I, Ken K, Mizuki S, et al. Dermoscopic features of pigmented Bowen's disease in a Japanese female mimicking malignant melanoma. *Dermatol Res Pract.* 2010;2010.
22. Hu C, Chiu H, Cheng G, et al. Dermoscopy as a diagnostic and follow-up tool for pigmented Bowen's disease on acral region. *Dermatol Surg.* 2008;34:1248–53.
23. Mun JH, Park JM, Song M, et al. The use of dermoscopy to monitor therapeutic response of Bowen's disease: A dermatoscopic pathologic study. *Br J Dermatol.* 2012;167:1382–85.
24. Hernàndez-Gil J, Fernandez-Pugnaire MA, Serrano-Falcòn C, et al. Clinical and dermoscopic features of pigmented Bowen's disease. *Actas Dermosifilogr.* 2008;99:419–27.

29 Nonpigmented skin lesions
Actinic keratosis and squamous cell carcinoma

Aimilios Lallas and Giuseppe Argenziano

Actinic keratosis (AK), Bowen's disease (BD), and invasive squamous cell carcinoma (SCC) represent malignant neoplasms of epidermal keratinocytes and are described under the umbrella term *keratinocyte skin cancer*.[1]

In the past, keratinocyte tumors were subdivided in premalignant or precursor lesions (AK), tumors of "intermediate" biologic nature (BD), and really malignant ones (invasive SCC).[2] Instead, keratinocyte skin cancer is today considered to represent an apparent continuum of neoplasms in different progression stages, with AK on the one edge and poorly differentiated SCC on the other.[3] This theory was initially based on the observation that invasive SCC rarely develops on healthy skin, typically being associated with preexisting AKs,[4–5] while further evidence was provided by genetic studies revealing that AK and SCC share common alterations in the p53 gene, bearing signature UV mutations in stem-cell-related clones.[1] The concept of field cancerization refers to the presence of genetically altered cell clones in normal-appearing skin contiguous to fields of neoplastic cells, which have the potential of clonal expansion and thus give rise to locally recurrent skin cancer.[6] The field cancerization concept is in line with the clinical observation that AKs usually develop as multiple lesions affecting an entire field of chronically actinic damaged skin. The latter theory is further supported by new observations from the use of topical immunomodulating drugs for the treatment of AKs. The application of low-dose imiquimod all over the surface of the affected field has been suggested to uncover subclinical AKs, by stimulating an inflammatory response derived by the dendritic cells, while unaffected areas do not react to the drug application.[7] Taking all this novel information into account, clinicians should be aware that although AK, BD, and SCC are traditionally described as separate entities, they represent different progression stages of one neoplasm, the keratinocyte skin cancer. The dermatoscopic features of BD are described in Chapter 28.

ACTINIC KERATOSIS

DEFINITION

Also known as solar keratosis or keratinocytic intraepidermal neoplasia, AK represents the earliest form of SCC. It is considered to be a precancerous lesion by some authors and *in situ* SCC by others.

EPIDEMIOLOGY/ETIOPATHOGENESIS

AK represents the most frequent carcinoma (*in situ*) in humans, and its incidence continues to rise.[8] However, the incidence of AK differs according to skin prototype and sun-exposure habits, being significantly higher in individuals with skin types I–III and in regions with a sunny climate. The highest frequency of AK has been reported in Australia, where it is estimated that 40%–60% of the population older than 40 years will develop AK. Overall, men are more commonly affected than women, with 34% of men and 18% of women over the age of 70 found to have AKs.[9]

Long-term UV light exposure plays the main role in the pathogenesis of AK. The risk of AK development directly correlates with the cumulative exposure to UV light and, accordingly, the frequency of AKs increases with age. Several medical procedures are known to induce AKs, especially those involving repeated iatrogenic exposure to UV radiation combined or not with psoralens, x-rays, or radioisotopes. Chronic immunosuppression is also known to represent an independent risk factor for development of nonmelanoma skin cancer, including AKs, while organ-transplanted patients have a 250-fold higher risk of developing AKs.[10–11] The reported risk of an individual AK to progress to invasive SCC varies from 0.1%–20%.[12–13] However, patients with multiple AKs have a 5-year cumulative probability of 14% to develop SCC, either within the AK or *de novo*, highlighting the need of regular follow-up.[12–13] As mentioned above, molecular and genetic studies suggest that AK represents the earliest form of SCC.

Clinical presentation/Diagnosis

AKs typically present clinically as erythematous hyperkeratotic macules, papules, or plaques on chronically sun-exposed areas such as the bald scalp, ears, face, forearms, and dorsum of the hands.[3] Several clinical subtypes have been described, including keratotic, verrucous, pigmented, atrophic and lichenoid forms, and cutaneous corn. Typically, lesions of different clinical subtypes are simultaneously present within a sun-damaged field.[14]

A clinical classification for grading AKs has been proposed. Grade I refers to slightly palpable AKs (better felt than seen); grade II includes AKs of moderate thickness (easily felt and seen); and grade III AKs are clinically obvious, very thick, and usually hyperkeratotic.[15]

Histopathologically, AKs are characterized by keratinocytic atypia, mitotic activity, hyperkeratosis, parakeratosis, dermal inflammatory infiltrate, and concomitant solar elastosis[16] (Figure 29.1). According to a proposed histomorphological classification, AKs may be subdivided into three grades, which correlate to specific clinical and dermatoscopic patterns.[17]

Dermatoscopy/Videodermatoscopy features

The three different clinical grades of AK at dermatoscopy correspond to three different patterns (Figures 29.2–29.4). Grade I AKs are typified

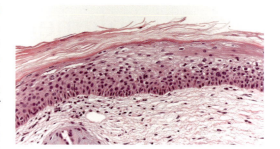

FIGURE 29.1 Histopathology of actinic keratosis. The epidermis is slightly thickened and shows focal parakeratosis. In the basal layer, keratinocytes nuclei are enlarged and hyperchromatic. An atypical mitotic figure is present in the center of the field.

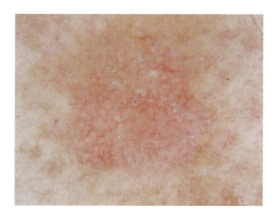

FIGURE 29.2 Dermatoscopy of grade I actinic keratosis typically revealing linear vessels surrounding the follicular openings, forming the so-called red pseudonetwork (×10).

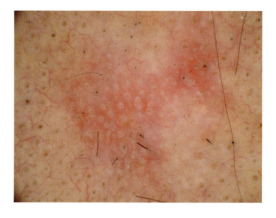

FIGURE 29.3 Dermatoscopy of grade II actinic keratosis characterized by a red background color, interrupted by the follicular openings that might be slightly dilated and filled with keratin plugs (×10).

Nonpigmented Skin Lesions

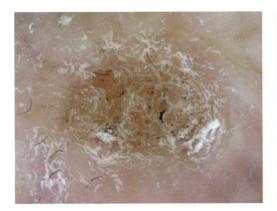

FIGURE 29.4 Dermatoscopy of grade III actinic keratosis. The compact hyperkeratosis, seen as an amorphous white-yellow mass, often impedes the visualization of underlying structures (×10).

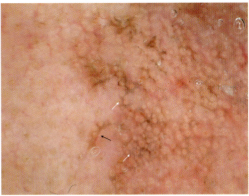

FIGURE 29.5 Dermatoscopy of pigmented actinic keratosis (PAK) might reveal gray color (white arrows), not allowing its discrimination from early lentigo maligna. However, the detection of a broken brown pseudonetwork (black arrow) and the presence of dilated follicular openings filled with keratin plugs are suggestive of the diagnosis of PAK (×10).

by a red pseudonetwork and white scales.[18] Grade II lesions typically reveals the so-called strawberry pattern, consisting of an erythematous background interrupted by white to yellow enlarged follicular openings with or without keratin plugs. In grade III AKs, the dense hyperkeratosis, seen as a white-yellow structureless area, often impedes the visualization of the follicular openings, which are typically filled with keratotic plugs.[18] The diagnostic sensitivity and specificity of dermatoscopy in the diagnosis of nonpigmented AK has been reported to reach 98% and 95%, respectively.[19]

Less often, AK may be slightly or heavily pigmented (pigmented AK-PAK), clinically presenting as a red-brownish or even brown macule. In such cases, clinical discrimination from solar lentigo (SL) or early lentigo maligna (LM) might be problematic.[20] When located on the face, dermatoscopy of PAK typically reveals the so-called pseudonetwork, consisting of a diffuse brown pigmentation interrupted by nonpigmented follicular openings (Figure 29.5), histopathologically corresponding to pigmented keratinocytes along the flattened dermo-epidermal junction of the facial skin. The latter dermatoscopic pattern can be also seen in SL and LM and, accordingly, the differential diagnosis of a pigmented facial macule relies on the detection of additional specific criteria.[20] Among the latter three entities, the dermatoscopic recognition of SL (which is considered a type of early seborrheic keratosis) is usually feasible, based on the absence of gray color and the detection of light-brown fingerprint areas, yellow opaque areas, milia-like cysts, a moth-eaten border, and a sharp demarcation.[20] Instead, the discrimination between PAK and LM may be very difficult, because both tumors have been reported to exhibit similar dermatoscopic features, including the established criteria of LM, such as asymmetrically pigmented follicular openings, rhomboidal structures, and gray dots or globules.[20] Some dermatoscopic clues have been suggested to indicate the diagnosis of PAK versus LM, including the presence of superficial scales, keratin plugs, sharp demarcation, and a broken-up pseudonetwork. In contrast, black blotches within the follicular opening occur at higher frequency in LM than in PAK. Nevertheless, histopathology is very often required to differentiate between LM and PAK.[21] Notably, the discrimination between the two entities may be even histopathologically difficult, when it is not clear whether the pigmented atypical cells in the basal layer are keratinocytes or melanocytes.[20]

In addition to significantly enhancing their recognition, preliminary data suggest a potential role of dermatoscopy in the monitoring of the treatment outcome of AKs.[22]

SQUAMOUS CELL CARCINOMA

Epidemiology/Etiopathogenesis

Primary cutaneous SCC is the second most common skin cancer, and its incidence has continuously risen over the last decades.[4] The majority (70%) of SCCs develop on the head and neck, with an additional 15% arising on the upper extremities.

UV radiation from sun exposure, occupational exposure, medical treatments (psoralen + UV-A [PUVA]), or tanning beds have been associated with the pathogenesis of SCC.[3–4] Immunosuppression has been also shown to significantly predispose to SCC development.[3]

The genetic background of SCC development includes UV-induced DNA mutations in the p53 tumor suppressor gene. This partially explains why SCC shows a predilection for fair-skinned individuals and chronically sun-exposed body sites.[23] Risk factors for SCC development include fair skin phototype, male gender, age over 40 years, and organ transplantation. Specifically, organ transplant recipients have a 65-fold increased risk of developing SCC compared to the general population. Interestingly, 22% of SCC in the latter group of patients arises on sun-protected body sites, such as the trunk or lower extremities.[3–4]

Clinical presentation/Diagnosis

Clinically, SCC usually presents as an indurated hyperkeratotic nodule with or without ulceration. Less often, SCC lacks signs of keratinization and manifests as an ulcer. The presence of AKs is usually evident on the neighboring and surrounding skin surface.[3]

Histopathologically, SCC is typified by the presence of nests of atypical keratinocytes, characterized by varying degrees of anaplasia and keratinization[24] (Figure 29.6). The tumor nests typically arise from the epidermis and extend into the dermis. Several histopathologic subtypes have been described, including spindle cell, pleomorphic, adenoid, acantholytic, and clear-cell SCC. Keratoacanthoma is also considered a well-differentiated subtype of SCC.[24]

Only about 2% of SCC is lethal, while the majority of the tumors have a generally favorable prognosis.[25] However, SCC can cause significant morbidity. This is because the majority of tumors

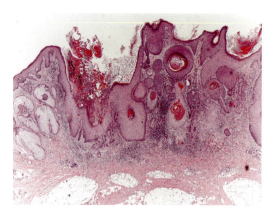

FIGURE 29.6 Histopathology of well-differentiated squamous cell carcinoma, made up of irregularly shaped, keratinizing nests deeply infiltrating the dermis.

arise on the head/neck area, where clear margins are difficult to obtain. The recurrence rate of SCC after surgery has been reported to range from 3.5%–28.0%.[23] The risk of recurrence depends on the patient's immune efficiency, as well as on factors related to the tumor, including body site, tumor size, invasion into the subcutaneous tissue, perineural involvement, and the grade of histopathologic differentiation.[23–26] While SCC has a 95% cure rate when detected and treated early, if neglected, it may cause local tissue destruction and metastasize, and in the latter case the prognosis is extremely poor. Furthermore, individuals with a primary SCC possess an 18% cumulative risk for developing a second tumor within 3 years, underlying the need for ongoing clinical monitoring.[27]

Dermatoscopy/Videodermatoscopy features

The dermatoscopic pattern of SCC depends on the degree of keratinization, which mirrors the grade of histopathologic differentiation.[3] Well-differentiated SCC is typified by a white predominant color, which can be attributed to several dermatoscopic structures, including white structureless areas, white circles, white halos, and white amorphous masses of keratin[3,18,28] (Figure 29.7). White structureless areas represent the most common but less specific feature. In contrast, white circles (or targetoid-appearing follicular openings) have been assessed as the

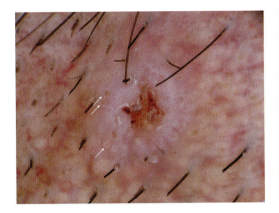

FIGURE 29.7 Dermatoscopy of well-differentiated squamous cell carcinoma showing a white predominant color; the presence of white circles (arrows) surrounding the follicular openings represents a highly specific clue (×10).

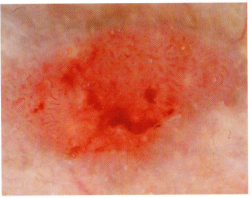

FIGURE 29.9 Dermatoscopy of poorly differentiated squamous cell carcinoma, displaying a red predominant color resulting from the presence of bleeding and/or numerous linear irregular vessels of small diameter in the absence of signs of keratinization (×10).

most specific feature of SCC when compared to other common nonpigmented skin tumors.[28] White halos and amorphous white keratin masses represent unmistakable markers of keratinization but are insufficient to predict a specific diagnosis. Vascular structures may be seen in well-differentiated SCC, usually as linear irregular or hairpin vessels of large diameter.[18] However, the quantity of vascular structures is usually low in well-differentiated SCC, with white structures typically predominating. A specific combination of central keratin masses surrounded by hairpin or linear irregular vessels distributed at the periphery of the tumor has been suggested to typify keratoacanthoma[18,28] (Figure 29.8).

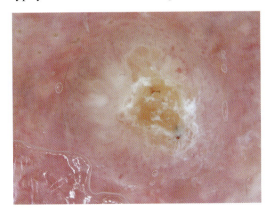

FIGURE 29.8 Typical dermatoscopic pattern of keratoacanthoma, consisting of a central amorphous white-yellow keratin mass and peripherally distributed linear irregular and/or hairpin vessels (×10).

The dermatoscopic morphology of poorly differentiated SCC significantly differs from the above described "white" pattern. Specifically, poorly differentiated SCC is clinically typified by a flat appearance and at dermatoscopy by a red predominant color, attributed to the absence of scaling and the presence of bleeding and/or dense vascularity[3] (Figure 29.9). The vessels' quantity is significantly correlated to the differentiation grade of SCC, because tumors displaying vessels in more than 50% of the lesion surface have a 30- to 120-fold increased possibility of being poorly differentiated. Vessels caliber also represents a significant predictor of differentiation grade, with a small caliber associated with poor differentiation.

By revealing vascular structures corresponding to the tumoral neo-angiogenesis, dermatoscopy may also be useful to differentiate between invasive SCC and *in-situ* variants (AK and BD).[18] Specifically, vascular patterns including dotted or glomerular vessels, hairpin vessels, and linear-irregular vessels occur at much higher frequency in SCC than in AK. Based on these morphologic observations, a progression model of AK developing toward SCC has been proposed. According to this model, progression from AK to invasive SCC is characterized by evident increase in vascularization, typified by the appearance of initially dotted or glomerular and later hairpin and linear vessels, along with a similar increase in the degree of keratinization.[18]

REFERENCES

1. Quatresooz P, Pierard-Franchimont C, Paquet P, et al. Crossroads between actinic keratosis and squamous cell carcinoma, and novel pharmacological issues. *Eur J Dermatol*. 2008;18:6–10.
2. MacKie RM, Quinn AG. Non-melanoma skin cancer and other epidermal skin tumours. In: *Rook's Textbook of Dermatology*. Burns T, Breathnach SM, Cox NH, Griffiths CEM, eds. 7th ed. Oxford: Blackwell, 2004: 36.1–36.39.
3. Lallas A, Argenziano G, Zendri E, et al. Update on non-melanoma skin cancer and the value of dermoscopy in its diagnosis and treatment monitoring. *Expert Rev Anticancer Ther*. 2013;13:541–58.
4. Alam M, Ratner D. Cutaneous squamous cell carcinoma. *N Engl J Med*. 2001;344:975–83.
5. Ackerman AB, Mones JM. Solar (actinic) keratosis is squamous cell carcinoma. *Br J Dermatol*. 2006;155:9–22.
6. Braakhuis BJM, Tabor MP, Kummer JA, et al. A genetic explanation of Slaughter's concept of field cancerization. *Cancer Res*. 2003;63:1727–30.
7. Stockfleth E, Gupta G, Peris K, et al. Reduction in lesions from Lmax: A new concept for assessing efficacy of field-directed therapy for actinic keratosis. Results with imiquimod 3.75%. *Eur J Dermatol*. 2014;24:23–27.
8. Memon AA, Tomenson JA, Bothwell J, Friedmann PS. Prevalence of solar damage and actinic keratosis in a Merseyside population. *Br J Dermatol*. 2000;142:1154–59.
9. Frost C, Williams G, Green A. High incidence and regression rates of solar keratoses in a Queensland community. *J Invest Dermatol*. 2000;115:273–77.
10. Brash DE, Ziegler A, Jonason AS, et al. Sunlight and sunburn in human skin cancer: p53, apoptosis, and tumor protection. *J Invest Dermatol Symp Proc*. 1996;1:136–42.
11. Ulrich C, Christophers E, Sterry W, et al. Skin diseases in organ transplant patients. *Hautarzt*. 2002;53:524–33.
12. Green A, Battistutta D. Incidence and determinants of skin cancer in a high-risk Australian population. *Int J Cancer*. 1990;46:356–61.
13. Glogau RG. The risk of progression to invasive disease. *J Am Acad Dermatol*. 2000;42:23–24.
14. Zalaudek I, Piana S, Moscarella E, et al. Morphologic grading and treatment of facial actinic keratosis. *Clin Dermatol*. 2014;32:80–87.
15. Rowert-Huber J, Patel MJ, Forschner T, et al. Actinic keratosis is an early *in situ* squamous cell carcinoma: A proposal for reclassification. *Br J Dermatol*. 2007;156:8–12.
16. Smoller BR. Squamous cell carcinoma: From precursor lesions to high-risk variants. *Mod Pathol*. 2006;19:S88–92.
17. Cockerell CJ. Histopathology of incipient intraepidermal squamous cell carcinoma ("actinic keratosis"). *J Am Acad Dermatol*. 2000;42:11–17.
18. Zalaudek I, Giacomel J, Schmid K, et al. Dermatoscopy of facial actinic keratosis, intraepidermal carcinoma, and invasive squamous cell carcinoma: A progression model. *J Am Acad Dermatol*. 2012;66:589–97.
19. Huerta-Brogeras M, Olmos O, Borbujo J et al. Validation of dermoscopy as a real-time noninvasive diagnostic imaging technique for actinic keratosis. *Arch Dermatol*. 2012;148:1159–64.
20. Lallas A, Argenziano G, Moscarella E, et al. Diagnosis and management of facial pigmented macules. *Clin Dermatol*. 2014;32:94–100.
21. Tschandl P, Rosendahl C, Kittler H. Dermatoscopy of flat pigmented facial lesions. *J Eur Acad Dermatol Venereol*. 2015;29(1):120–27.
22. Kaçar N, Sanli B, Zalaudek I, et al. Dermatoscopy for monitoring treatment of actinic keratosis with imiquimod. *Clin Exp Dermatol*. 2012;37:567–69.
23. Chren MM, Linos E, Torres JS, et al. Tumor recurrence after treatment of cutaneous basal cell carcinoma and squamous cell carcinoma. *J Invest Dermatol*. 2013;133:1188–96.
24. Cassarino DS, Derienzo DP, Barr RJ. Cutaneous squamous cell carcinoma: A comprehensive clinicopathologic classification. Part one. *J Cutan Pathol*. 2006;33:191–206.
25. Schmilts CD, Karia PS, Carter JB, et al. Factors predictive of recurrence and death from cutaneous squamous cell carcinoma: A 10-year, single-institution cohort study. *JAMA Dermatol*. 2013;149:541–47.
26. Brinkman JN, Haider E, van der Holt B, et al. The effect of differentiation grade of cutaneous squamous cell carcinoma on excision margins,

local recurrence, metastasis, and patient survival: A retrospective follow-up study. *Ann Plast Surg.* 2014 Jan. 7 (Epub).
27. Frankel DH, Hanusa BH, Zitelli JA. New primary nonmelanoma skin cancer in patients with a history of squamous cell carcinoma of the skin: Implications and recommendations for follow-up. *J Am Acad Dermatol.* 1992;26:720–26.
28. Rosendahl C, Cameron A, Argenziano G, et al. Dermoscopy of squamous cell carcinoma and keratoacanthoma. *Arch Dermatol.* 2012;148:1386–92.

30 Capillary malformations

Francisco Vázquez-López and Begoña García-García

DEFINITION

Vascular anomalies may be classified into vascular tumors (presence of cellular proliferation) and vascular malformations (VMs) (aberrations in morphogenesis with ectasia of vessels). VMs are classified (according to the predominant vessel type and flow characteristic on Doppler ultrasound or magnetic resonance imaging) on slow-flow lesions (including venous, capillary, or lymphatic VMs) and fast-flow lesions (including arteriovenous malformations with clinically significant arteriovenous shunting).[1–6]

Capillary malformations (CMs) represent the most common VMs and include port-wine stains (PWSs) as well as telangiectasias.[1–6]

EPIDEMIOLOGY/ETIOPATHOGENESIS

CMs affect 0.3%–0.5% of newborns. Their origin is unclear, possibly being a result of a vascular developmental or innervation defect. Most cases are congenital and sporadic, but acquired and familial cases (related to mutation in the RASA1 gene)[7–8] have been reported. CMs may be syndromic, within the context of Sturge-Weber syndrome (SWS) or not: in both cases, a mutation in GNAQ gen (chromosome 9q21) has been suggested.[9]

CLINICAL PRESENTATION/DIAGNOSIS

CMs tend to be present at birth and grow with age. They are characterized by ectatic vessels with flattened endothelium; most of them are situated in the papillary dermis and upper part of the reticular dermis, but they may be located deeper (Figure 30.1). Clinically, they are initially macular, but growth is marked by thickening and increased nodularity in time. The color varies from pink to red to deep purple. CMs may be localized or have a segmental distribution (such as the typical sensory trigeminal nerve distribution of lesions located on the head and neck). Facial CMs characteristically darken and become more violaceous with age, whereas lesions on the trunk and limbs may fade to a lighter pink. CMs on the limbs may further be associated with hypertrophy of underlying bone and soft tissue as well as deeper malformations of larger vessels (Klippel-Trenaunay and Parkes Weber syndromes).[1–6]

CMs must be evaluated by multidisciplinary teams in severe cases. The classification and management of patients may be difficult and must consider variables such as family history, genetics, age of appearance, age of the patient at treatment, evolution, hormonal aggravation factors, and presence of syndromic signs. Essential clinical data are color (blue, pink, red, purplish), thickness (macular or elevated), size, location and distribution (isolated, segmental), palpation (firm or compressible, thrill), temperature, and pain.

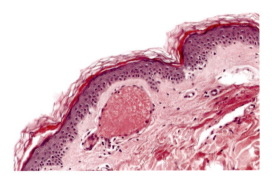

FIGURE 30.1 Histopathologically, capillary malformations are characterized by ectatic vessels with flattened endothelium, most of them situated in the papillary dermis and upper part of the reticular dermis.

DERMATOSCOPY/VIDEODERMATOSCOPY FEATURES

By means of dermatoscopy, a better understanding of the morphology of the vessels involved in CMs can be easily obtained, revealing vascular structures not visible during standard visual inspection. Dermatoscopy may be performed with nonpolarized or polarized devices, with filters for glare reduction. Standard magnification of handheld dermatoscopes is ×10; it may be increased by means of the digital zoom of a photocamera, but the image quality decreases. Videodermatoscope units and stereomicroscopes offering greater magnifications and resolution are also available.

Both vascular (round and linear vessels)[10–13] and nonvascular structures (gray-whitish veil) have been described in CMs with videodermatoscopy, stereomicroscopy, and dermatoscopy.[10–15] According to most studies, CMs have been classified into predominantly type 1 (superficial) and type 2 (deep) patterns.[11] In addition, a type 3 and a mixed and undefined pattern have also been described[14–15] (Figures 30.2–30.8, Table 30.1). A correlation between clinical, histological, and dermatoscopic parameters of CMs has been found by some authors.[16–17] Type 1 vessels are round to oval, sharp, red structures with a variable size (dotted, pint-pointed, or globular) (Figures 30.2–30.4). They have been

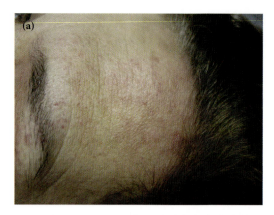

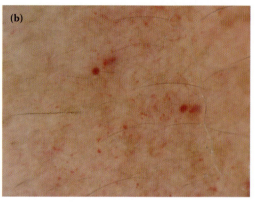

FIGURE 30.2 (a) Flat, partially treated, long-standing capillary malformation of the forehead. (b) Dermatoscopy revealing a type 1, superficial pattern, characterized by scattered red, rounded, ectatic vessels of variable size (×10).

TABLE 30.1
Dermatoscopic patterns of CMs

Dermatoscopic Pattern	Morphology	Histopathological Correlation	Response to Laser Treatment
• Type 1 vessels	• Red, round dots/globules	• Ectatic papillary vessels • Superficial vessels	Best response
• Type 2 vessels	• Reticular linear vessels	• Ectatic horizontal subpapillary plexus • Deeper vessels	Lower response
• Type 3 vessels	• Round vessels directly connected to linear vessels	• Sacular ectasias of the horizontal plexus • Deeper vessels in long-standing lesions	Lower response
• Mixed, undefined patterns	• Variable	• Variable	Unknown
• Gray-whitish veil	• Obscured vessels	• Deeper vessels	Lower response

Capillary Malformations

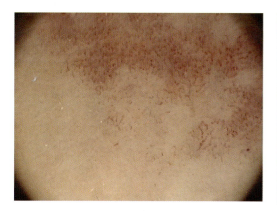

FIGURE 30.3 Dermatoscopy of capillary malformation showing type 1, round capillaries in greater number. The contrast with the surrounding normal skin is easily visible (×10).

correlated to ectatic capillary loops of the papillae,[11] measuring from 0.3 to 0.4 mm in diameter.[15] Type 2 vessels are red linear vessels, variable in tortuousity, width, length, and sharpness, forming irregular networks (Figures 30.5–30.7). They have been correlated to the deeper horizontal subepidermal vascular plexus[11] and sized from 0.08 to 0.1 mm in width.[15] They seem to present higher blood flow compared with the Type 1 pattern.[15] Type 3 vessels have been reported[15] but not yet confirmed. They represent round (sacular, glomerular) structures directly connected

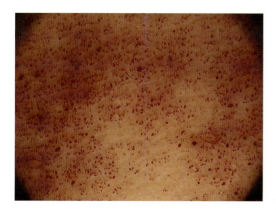

FIGURE 30.4 Dermatoscopy of capillary malformation showing numerous type 1 round vessels, disclosing a variable size (dotted, globular, and similar to lagoons) (×10).

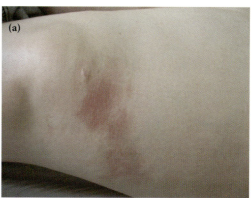

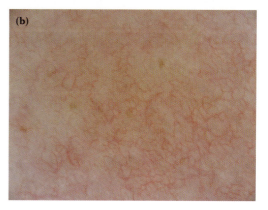

FIGURE 30.5 (a) Capillary malformation located on the thigh. (b) Dermatoscopy revealing a type 2 vascular pattern: tortuous, thin, linear vessels configured in an irregular network are evident (×10).

with the horizontal plexus. It has been hypothesized that they result from an "aneurismatic" enlargement of the horizontal plexus over time and have been related to age and arterial hypertension. Type 1 round vessels of CMs may be dotted or globular. The largest globules resemble the "red lagoons" of hemangiomas, which are red, sharply demarcated, varying in size, oval to round structures, clustered or loosely scattered. Lagoons of hemangiomas are secondary to both proliferation and ectasia of the vessels involved; round vessels of CMs present only vascular dilatation (Figures 30.9–30.12). Finally, a grayish-white veil has been reported associated to and hiding the deeper vessels of the lower reticular dermis.[14]

Dermatoscopy has been demonstrated to be useful for predicting response of CMs to laser

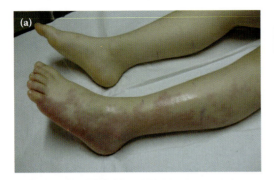

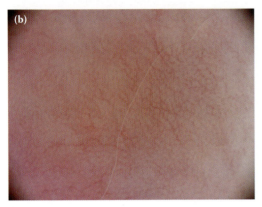

FIGURE 30.6 (a) Capillary malformation located on the leg. (b) Dermatoscopy revealing a predominant type 2 vascular pattern (linear vessels) but also scattered dotted, type 1 vessels and type 3 sacular vessels (×10).

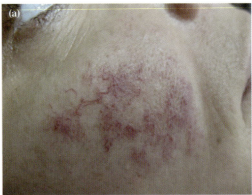

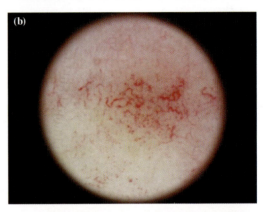

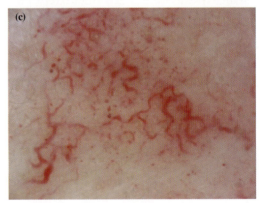

FIGURE 30.7 (a) Capillary malformation located on the cheek previously treated with laser (blanched areas are easily visible). (b) Dermatoscopy revealing a mixed pattern with linear, tortuous, short, and arboriform vessels and also round, globular vessels (×10). (c) Dermatoscopy at higher magnification (digital zoom): tortuous linear vessels and globular vessels are demonstrated herein despite the previous therapy.

treatment, in particular to pulsed dye laser. Several factors influencing this response have been reported[16–22] (Table 30.2). According to clinical data, for example, purple and red lesions respond better than the pink ones.[18–19] A number of histological studies have established the importance of capillary depth and diameter in determining the response of CMs to laser treatments: deeper vessels with a small diameter respond less well.[20–21] Dermatoscopy providing data on the depth of the vessels involved in CMs adds useful prognostic information. The presence of type 2 vessels,[10–11,15] gray-whitish veil,[14] and type 3 vessels[15] have been related to less response to treatment, whereas type 1 superficial vessels have been related to a better response. A videomicroscope able to

TABLE 30.2
Factors influencing the response of CMs to laser treatment

1. **Clinical data:** color, location, size of VM, age of patients
2. **Dermatoscopic data:** type of vessels, gray-whitish veil
3. **Histological data:** depth and diameter of the capillaries of CM
4. **Other data:** competing chromophores; skin thickness, blood flow

determine morphology, depth, and diameter of capillaries (depth-measuring videomicroscope, DMV) has been developed and applied for evaluating CMs.[16–17] This tool is similar to a traditional videomicroscopic unit but allows a recording of individual capillaries to be imaged and their depth and diameter to be calculated. The results obtained with DMV confirm the previous histological results that the small, deeply located vessels are more resistant to the laser treatment.

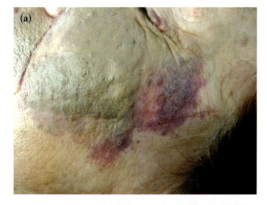

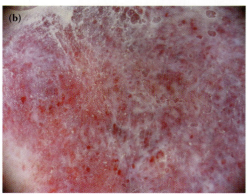

FIGURE 30.8 (a) Longstanding capillary malformation of the face, partially masked by a cosmetic camouflage and partially treated with electrodessication. At this phase, lesions may become darker and violaceous, thicker, and may develop blebs. (b) Dermatoscopy revealing an undefined pattern, with a deep purplish background, round vascular structures, and a delicate whitish network (×10).

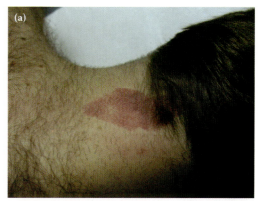

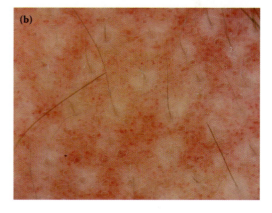

FIGURE 30.9 (a) Patient with a prominent mid-line "salmon patch" capillary malformation of the neck. (b) Dermatoscopy showing a homogeneous type 1 globular vascular patter devoid of linear vessels.

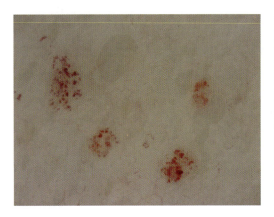

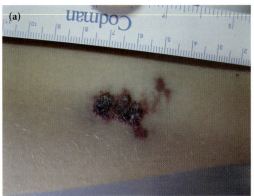

FIGURE 30.10 Dermatoscopy of acquired hemangioma, characterized by lagoons or lacunae, which are red to blue-red or blue-black to maroon, round to oval, sharp structures, either tightly clustered or loosely scattered throughout the lesion.

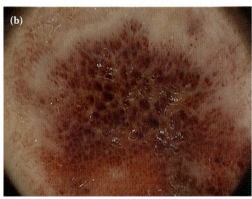

In conclusion, dermatoscopy, in conjunction with clinical examination, improves the understanding of the morphology of the vessels of CMs by revealing subclinical insights with a prognostic significance. Moreover, it may be speculated that in the future, dermatoscopy may facilitate the development of newer lasers to treat CMs more efficiently as pulse duration and wavelength could be matched to measured vessel diameter and depth, respectively.

FIGURE 30.12 (a) Patient with a mixed vascular malformation on the arm with prominent deep component. (b) Dermatoscopy showing tightly clustered red globular vessels and blue lagoons, which are related to the vessel ectasia and not to vascular proliferation.

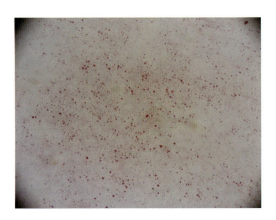

FIGURE 30.11 Dermatoscopy of acquired angioma serpiginosum: multiple scattered, sharp lagoons.

REFERENCES

1. Dompmartin A. Classification of vascular anomalies. *Ann Dermatol Venereol.* 2013:140:337–39.
2. Barreau M, Dompmartin A. Non-syndromic cutaneous vascular malformations. *Ann Dermatol Venereol.* 2014;141:56–67.
3. Happle R. What is a capillary malformation? *J Am Acad Dermatol.* 2008;59:1077–79.
4. Garzon MC, Huang JT, Enjolras O, Frieden IJ. Vascular malformations: Part I. *J Am Acad Dermatol.* 2007;56:353–70.
5. Meghan FS, Glick SA, Hirsch RJ. Laser treatment of pediatric vascular lesions: Port wine stains and hemangiomas. *J Am Acad Dermatol.* 2008;58:261–85.

6. Aboytalebi A, Jessup CJ, North PE, Mihm MC Jr. Histopathology of vascular anomalies. *Facial Plast Surg.* 2012;28:545–53.
7. Eerola I, Boon LM, Watanabe S, et al. Locus for susceptibility for familial capillary malformation ("port-wine stain") maps to 5q. *Eur J Hum Genet.* 2002;10:375–80.
8. Hershkovitz D, Bercovich D, Sprecher E, Lapidot M. RASA1 mutations may cause hereditary capillary malformations without arteriovenous malformations. *Br J Dermatol.* 2008;158:1035–40.
9. Shirley MD, Tang H, Gallione CJ, et al. Sturge-Weber syndrome and port-wine stains caused by somatic mutations in GNAQ. *N Engl J Med.* 2013;23;368:1971–79.
10. Motley RJ, Lanigan SW, Katugampola GA. Videomicroscopy predicts outcome in treatment of port-wine stains. *Arch Dermatol.* 1997;133:921–22.
11. Eubanks LE, McBurney EI. Videomicroscopy of port-wine stains: Correlation of location and depth of lesion. *J Am Acad Dermatol.* 2003;48:984–85.
12. Vázquez-López F, Manjón-Haces JA, Vázquez-López AC, Pérez-Oliva N. The handheld dermatoscope improves the clinical evaluation of port-wine stains. *J Am Acad Dermatol.* 2003;48:984–85.
13. Sevila A, Nagore E, Botella-Estrada R, et al. Videomicroscopy of venular malformations (port-wine stain type): prediction of response to pulsed dye laser. *Pediatr Dermatol.* 2004;21:589–96.
14. Procaccini EM, Argenziano G, Staibano S, et al. Epiluminescence microscopy for port-wine stains: Pretreatment evaluation. *Dermatology.* 2001;203:329–32.
15. Bencini PL, Cazzaniga S, Galimberti MG, et al. Variables affecting clinical response to treatment of facial port-wine stains by flash lamp-pumped pulsed dye laser: The importance of looking beyond the skin. *Lasers Med Sci.* 2014;29:1365–70.
16. Sivarajan V, Mackay IR The depth measuring videomicroscope (DMV): A noninvasive tool for the assessment of capillary vascular malformations. *Lasers Surg Med.* 2004;34:193–97.
17. Sivarajan V, MacKay IR. The relationship between location, color, and vessel structure within capillary vascular malformations. *Ann Plast Surg.* 2004;53:378–81.
18. Renfro L, Geronemus RG. Anatomical differences of port-wine stains in response to treatment with the pulsed dye laser. *Arch Dermatol.* 1993;129:182–88.
19. Nguyen CM, Yohn JJ, Huff C, et al. Facial port wine stains in childhood: Prediction of the rate of improvement as a function of the age of the patient, size and location of the port wine stain and the number of treatments with the pulsed dye (585 nm) laser. *Br J Dermatol.* 1998;138:821–25.
20. Onizuka K, Tsuneda K, Shibata Y, et al. Efficacy of flashlamp-pumped pulsed dye laser therapy for port wine stains: Clinical assessment and histopathological characteristics. *Br J Plast Surg.* 1995;48:271–79.
21. Fiskerstrand EJ, Svaasand LO, Kopstad G, et al. Laser treatment of port wine stains: Therapeutic outcome in relation to morphological parameters. *Br J Dermatol.* 1996;134:1039–43.
22. Nagore E, Requena C, Sevila A, et al. Thickness of healthy and affected skin of children with port wine stains: Potential repercussions on response to pulsed dye laser treatment. *Dermatol Surg.* 2004;30:1457–61.

31 Miscellaneous disorders

Enzo Errichetti, Giuseppe Stinco, Anna Elisa Verzì, Francesco Lacarrubba, Salvatore Ferraro, Cecilia Santagati, and Giuseppe Micali

The diagnosis of several disorders in addition to those covered in previous chapters may be supported by dermatoscopy. These include inflammatory disorders (lichen sclerosus, morphea, lichen nitidus), genodermatoses (Darier's disease), genital growths (Fordyce's spots, pearly penile papules, vestibular papillae), and other conditions (Kaposi's sarcoma, cutaneous mastocytosis, milia).

LICHEN SCLEROSUS

Definition

Lichen sclerosus (LS) is a chronic inflammatory dermatosis that results in white plaques.

Epidemiology/Etiopathogenesis

LS is a common disease that primarily involves the anogenital area (85% of cases), but extragenital lesions (15% of cases) can also occur. It is five times more prevalent in women than men.[1–2] The causes of LS are unknown, but some studies showed a significant correlation with the presence of antibodies against the extracellular matrix protein-1, thus supporting a possible autoimmune pathogenesis;[3] a genetic component was also hypothesized.[1–2]

Clinical presentation/Diagnosis

Clinically, LS presents with whitish, polygonal papules coalescing into plaques of varying size and shape (Figure 31.1a). Fissures, telangiectasias, purpura, erythema, and erosions may be seen in both anogenital and extragenital lesions, while follicular plugs are generally evident only in the active/early phase of extragenital LS. Over the time, the latter results in smooth, atrophic, porcelain-white lesions, while anogenital LS may lead to destructive scarring sequelae. Unlike extragenital LS, which is asymptomatic, anogenital lesions are frequently associated with itching, soreness, dyspareunia, dysuria, discomfort with defecation, and/or genital bleeding.[1–2]

Early LS is histologically characterized by hyperkeratosis and hypergranulosis of the adnexal structures, mild acanthosis, focal basement membrane thickening, subepithelial edema, homogenized collagen, and dilated blood vessels immediately under the basement membrane, while more advanced LS lesions typically show epidermal atrophy with flattening of the rete ridges, vacuolar interface changes, loss of elastic fibers, and hyalinization of the lamina propria with an underlying lymphocytic infiltrate.[2]

Dermatoscopy/Videodermatoscopy features

The dermatoscopic aspect of LS varies according to the localization and clinicopathological evolution of the lesions.[4] The main features of both anogenital and extragenital LS include whitish patches and linear branching vessels.[5–6] Moreover, dotted vessels and comedo-like openings are also frequently seen in anogenital and early extragenital lesions, respectively[4–7] (Figure 31.1b). Less commonly, anogenital LS may present erosions, comedo-like openings, scales, and chrysalis structures, while extragenital LS may show fibrotic beams, scales, chrysalis structures, gray dots, pigment network-like structures, and nonbranching vessels (comma-like, hairpin, and dotted).[5–6] According to the literature, comedo-like openings and whitish patches, histologically corresponding, respectively, to follicular plugging and epidermal atrophy, are considered two dermatoscopic clues for distinguishing extragenital LS from morphea.[5,7]

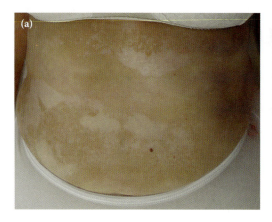
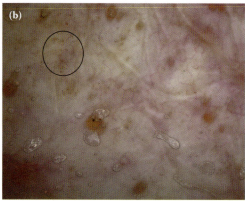

FIGURE 31.1 (a) Lichen sclerosus of the abdomen: white, polygonal papules coalescing into wide plaques. (b) Dermatoscopy showing three main features: whitish patches, linear branching vessels, and yellowish comedo-like openings; dotted vessels are also evident (circle) (×10).

MORPHEA

DEFINITION

Morphea (or localized scleroderma) is a self-limited or chronically relapsing, connective tissue disorder involving skin and subcutaneous tissue.

EPIDEMIOLOGY/ETIOPATHOGENESIS

Morphea is relatively rare and three times more common in women than in men.[8–9] The etiopathogenesis of morphea is poorly understood, but an autoimmune mechanism has been speculated based on the high frequency of autoantibody formation and personal and/or familial history of autoimmune disease in affected patients.[10] While there are no conclusive data, several factors have been related to the development of morphea, including radiation, infections, surgery, insect bites, and intramuscular injections.[8]

CLINICAL PRESENTATION/DIAGNOSIS

Classically, morphea begins as one or more erythematous patches evolving into sclerotic plaques with an ivory white-colored center and erythematous-to-violaceous active border (lilac ring) (Figure 31.2a). Over the time, the

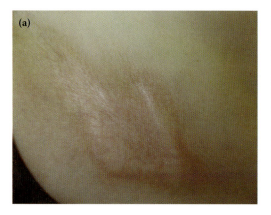
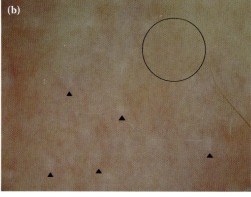

FIGURE 31.2 Morphea. (a) Sclerotic plaques with an ivory white-colored center and brownish border; erythema and telangiectasias are also evident (activity signs). (b) Dermatoscopy showing whitish beams (arrowheads) and linear branching vessels; a few brownish lines, some of which intersect to form a network-like structure (circle), are also evident (×10).

Miscellaneous Disorders

sclerotic plaque softens and becomes atrophic with hypo- or hyperpigmentation; there is also loss of hair follicles and sweat glands. Morphea includes several subtypes such as morphea in plaque, generalized, bullous, linear, and deep.[8] Histologically, active lesions of morphea are characterized by a perivascular and interstitial infiltrate of lymphocytes admixed with plasma cells and occasional eosinophils in the reticular dermis and/or subcutaneous tissues; initial thickening of collagen bundles is also evident. In the late sclerotic stage, the inflammatory infiltrate typically disappears and collagen bundles become thick, closely packed, and hyalinized; a paucity of blood vessels is seen, and adnexal structures are progressively lost.[11]

Dermatoscopy/Videodermatoscopy features

Dermatoscopy of morphea typically shows accentuated whitish beams, histologically corresponding to dermal sclerosis, crossed by linear branching vessels;[5,9] pigment network-like structures are also frequently evident[5] (Figure 31.2b). Importantly, comedo-like openings and whitish patches, two findings frequently detectable in lichen sclerosus, may also be seen less commonly in morphea.[5] However, according to one study, the presence of such features would be more indicative of a diagnosis of lichen sclerosus, while the detection of fibrotic beams would be more characteristic of morphea.[5] Interestingly, some authors have suggested using dermatoscopy in therapeutic monitoring because it would allow an accurate assessment of decreases in the fibrotic process (whitish beams) and the regression of neovessels (branching vessels) typical of morphea.[5]

LICHEN NITIDUS

Definition

Lichen nitidus (LN) is an idiopathic benign chronic dermatosis first described by Pinkus in 1901.[12]

Epidemiology/Etiopathogenesis

LN is rare, with an estimated incidence of about 0.3 cases/100,000 population. It affects mainly children and young adults. The etiology is unknown.

Clinical presentation/Diagnosis

Clinically, LN typically presents as minute (1–2 mm), flesh-colored or hypopigmented, asymptomatic shiny papules (Figure 31.3a). Several unusual variants have also been reported, including actinic, perforating, keratodermic, vesicular, and purpuric/hemorrhagic forms. The Koebner phenomenon may be observed, and it is thought to be responsible for linear arrangement of the lesions revealed in some cases.[12–13] The most commonly involved sites include the abdomen, chest, extremities, and genitalia (especially in men), but atypical localizations such as mucous membranes, nails, palms, and soles have also been reported.[12] LN

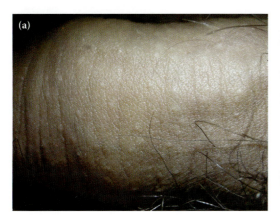
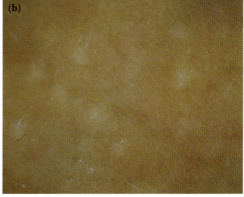

FIGURE 31.3 Lichen nitidus. (a) Minute, flesh-colored papules restricted to the foreskin. (b) Dermatoscopy showing several whitish homogeneous clouds, each one corresponding to a papule (×10).

is histologically characterized by a lympho-histiocytic inflammatory cell infiltrate (which may be granulomatous) that lies immediately below the thinned epidermis and is enveloped by bordering elongated rete ridges. Basal cell hydropic degeneration and central parakeratosis without hypergranulosis may also be present.[12] The diagnosis of LN is mainly clinical, based on its distinctive features.[13] However, particularly when lesions are localized to genitalia, LN may easily be misdiagnosed with consequent inappropriate treatments. The main differential diagnoses of genital LN are genital warts and molluscum contagiosum.

Dermatoscopy/Videodermatoscopy features

LN is characterized at dermatoscopy by whitish homogeneous clouds (one for each papule) (Figure 31.3b), histologically corresponding to the well-delimited inflammatory cell infiltrate just below the epidermis. Such dermatoscopic pattern is quite different from that of genital warts and molluscum contagiosum.[14–15]

DARIER'S DISEASE

Definition

Darier's disease (DD), also known as keratosis follicularis, is a rare autosomal dominant acantholytic disorder.

Epidemiology/Etiopathogenesis

The prevalence of DD has been estimated to range from 1/30,000 to 1/100,000. It is due to a mutations in the gene ATP2A2, which encodes the sarcoplasmic/endoplasmic reticulum Ca^{2+}-ATP isoform 2 protein (SERCA2), a pump transporting Ca^{2+} from the cytosol to the lumen of the endoplasmic reticulum. While most patients with DD have a family history of the disease, spontaneous mutations are not infrequent; the disease generally appears between the ages of 6 and 20 years.[16]

Clinical presentation/Diagnosis

Clinically, DD is characterized by discrete, greasy, hyperkeratotic, skin-colored, reddish-brown or yellowish-brown papules mainly located in seborrheic areas and skin creases (including the axillae, groins, and perineum) (Figure 31.4a); they may sometimes coalesce into crusted plaques. Symptoms include itch, malodor, and pain. Nail abnormalities, acral lesions, and mucous membrane changes are often present and may be the first signs of disease. Clinical variants include erosive, vesiculobullous, hyperkeratotic, comedonal, freckled "Groveroid," hypopigmented, and segmental forms.[16] The diagnosis is based on histological examination that shows downgrowths of narrow cords of keratinocytes, suprabasal

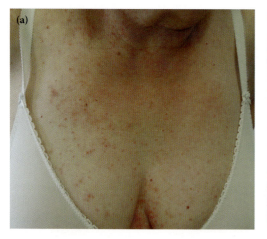
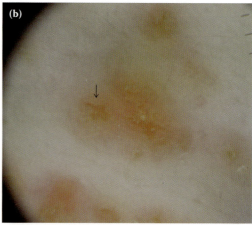

FIGURE 31.4 Darier diseases. (a) Several greasy, hyperkeratotic, reddish-brown papules on the décolleté area. (b) Dermatoscopy showing reddish-brownish papules with superficial indentations and tan-colored scaly areas; one papule presents a star-like aspect (arrow) (×10).

acantholysis with suprabasal clefts, dyskeratosis, and hyperkeratosis; apoptosis resulting in rounded eosinophilic dyskeratotic cells in the epidermis (corps ronds) and flattened parakeratotic cells in the horny layer (grains) may also be evident.[16–17]

Dermatoscopy/Videodermatoscopy

In a study on five patients the so-called giant pseudocomedones were the main dermatoscopic features of DD; they consisted of oval openings filled with a large yellow/brown keratotic plug, with raised or flat borders. The vascular pattern was reported as being variable, comprising erythema, dotted vessels, and linear vessels.[17] In another study of 11 patients, the most common dermatoscopic pattern consisted of a centrally located polygonal, star-like, or roundish-oval shaped yellowish/brownish area surrounded by a more or less thin whitish halo, overlying a pinkish homogeneous structureless area. (Figure 31.4b).[18] The star-like structures also may be seen in other dermatological conditions, including Dowling-Degos disease, acantholytic dyskeratotic acanthoma, and, particularly, Grover's disease.[19] The dermatoscopic overlap between DD and Grover's disease might be explained by their possible clinicopathological similarity.[16]

FORDYCE'S SPOTS OF THE PENILE SHAFT

Definition

Fordyce's spots of the penile shaft represent ectopic sebaceous glands.

Epidemiology/Etiopathogenesis

Fordyce's spots are very common, being present in about one-third of adult men, and represent normal variants of the skin of the penile shaft, especially on the ventral surface.

Clinical Presentation/Diagnosis

Clinically, Fordyce's spots of the penile shaft appear as symmetrical yellowish papules 1–2 mm in diameter (Figure 31.5a). Diagnosis is generally clinical, but sometimes they may be misdiagnosed with other genital growths, such as molluscum contagiosum, genital warts, or lymphangiomas.[20]

Dermatoscopy/Videodermatoscopy features

Fordyce's spots of the penile shaft show at dermatoscopy a typical vascular "garland-like" aspect, whose "bows" seem to wind around yellowish bunch-like lobules without crossing them (Figure 31.5b).[20] Histologically, the yellowish bunches correlate with the presence of groups of sebaceous lobules.

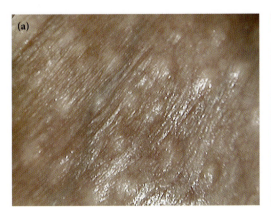
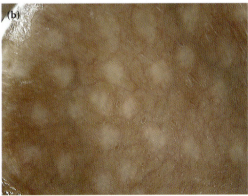

FIGURE 31.5 Fordyce's spots. (a) Multiple small yellowish papules of the penile shaft. (b) Dermatoscopy showing "swallow's nests" or "bottle-like" formations, containing a milky-white ovoid material and surrounded by wreath-like, non-arborizing vessels (×10).

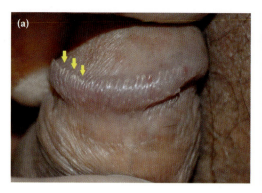 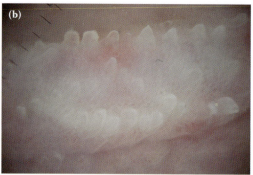

FIGURE 31.6 Pearly penile papules. (a) Symmetrical projections located circumferentially around the corona of the glans penis (arrows). (b) Dermatoscopy showing a characteristic whitish pink grape-like appearance (×10).

PEARLY PENILE PAPULES AND VESTIBULAR PAPILLAE

Definition

Pearly penile papules (PPP) (synonyms: Tyson glands, hirsutoid papillomas, papilla in the corona glandis, hirsutis papillary corona of the penis, pink pearly papules) are asymptomatic angiofibromas, typically distributed on the glans.[21]

Vestibular papillae (VP) are considered an anatomical variant of the vestibular mucosa. There is no causal association with HPV infection, and it is likely that this condition is the female counterpart of male PPP.[22]

Epidemiology/Etiopathogenesis

PPP occur most frequently in the second and third decades, more commonly in African-American and circumcised men. VP has a prevalence rate between 1% and 33%.

Clinical presentation/Diagnosis

PPP are typically asymptomatic, flesh-colored to pearly, 1–2 mm, smooth or dome-shaped papules located circumferentially around the corona and sulcus of the glans penis (Figure 31.6a). The histologic findings are those of angiofibromas.

Clinically, VP present as soft, 1–2 mm in diameter, flesh-colored, pearly, and filiform lesions, which may be symmetrical or linear[23] (Figure 31.7a). Although VP are usually asymptomatic, they may be associated with itching, pain, burning, or dyspareunia.[24] They may involve the labia minora and the introitus vaginae to a variable extent.[24] If a large number of papillae cover the entire surface of the labia

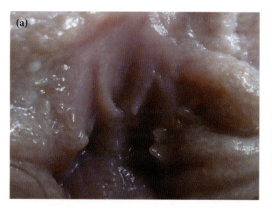 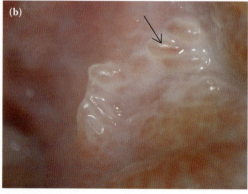

FIGURE 31.7 Vestibular papillae. (a) Several flesh-colored, pearly, and filiform lesions of 1–2 mm in diameter involving the introitus vaginae. (b) Dermatoscopy showing several filiform projections, each of which presents a separate base and a regular vascular axis (arrow) (×20).

minora in a symmetric fashion, the condition is referred to as vestibular papillomatosis.[46] VP is histologically characterized by finger-like protrusions of a loose connective tissue covered by normal vulvar epithelium.

Both PPP and VP are often misinterpreted as genital warts.[21–23]

Dermatoscopy/Videodermatoscopy features

The dermatoscopic pattern of PPP shows a characteristic whitish pink cobblestone or grape-like appearance in a few rows with central dotted or comma-like vessels in each papule (Figure 31.6b). The papules are further surrounded by crescent-shaped whitish structures.[20–21]

Dermatoscopy may facilitate the recognition of VP by magnifying the bases of the individual filiform projections, which typically remain separate, and showing a regular vascular axis[24] (Figure 31.7b). Such peculiar dermatoscopic aspect is quite different from that of condyloma acuminata, which notoriously consists of multiple whitish, irregular projections presenting conglomerate vascular structures and tapering ends arising from a common base.[24]

KAPOSI'S SARCOMA

Definition

Kaposi's sarcoma (KS) is a low-grade angioproliferative disorder of vascular endothelium, primarily affecting mucocutaneous tissues with the potential to involve viscera.[25] Four clinical variants have been recognized: classic, African (endemic), acquired immunodeficiency syndrome-associated epidemic, and iatrogenic. Each form has its own natural history, site of predilection, and prognosis.[26]

Epidemiology/Etiopathogenesis

The annual incidence of classic KS in the United States is estimated to be 0.02%–0.06% of all malignant tumors. The iatrogenic KS has been increasing in incidence among immunosuppressed patients, while the prevalence of KS in patients infected with HIV has declined throughout the epidemic.[27] Males are most commonly affected. All forms of KS have a common viral etiology by Kaposi sarcoma herpes virus/human herpes virus-8 (KSHV/HHV-8), and the differences among them are due to the involvement of various cofactors (genetic, immunologic, and environmental).[28]

Clinical presentation/Diagnosis

KS presents as either single or multiple, variably colored (purplish-red) and distributed macules, nodules, bullae, and plaques depending on the clinical variant and the stage of the disease (Figure 31.8a). Lesions are most commonly located on the lower extremities, especially the ankles and feet, whereas in people with AIDS-associated KS, the trunk is often involved. The clinical diagnosis of single KS lesions may be difficult, as they may resemble other cutaneous manifestations such as hemangioma, angiokeratoma, pyogenic granuloma, targetoid hemosiderotic hemangioma, angiosarcoma, fibrous histiocytoma, granuloma annulare, and melanocytic nevus.[29] The final diagnosis of KS relies

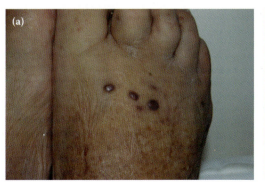
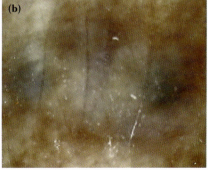

FIGURE 31.8 Kaposi's sarcoma. (a) Multiple purplish-red macules and nodules of the foot. (b) Dermatoscopy showing the typical "rainbow" pattern (×10).

on histopathology that shows a proliferation of spindle cells and endothelial cells to form closely arranged slit-like vascular spaces.

Dermatoscopy/Videodermatoscopy features

Under dermatoscopy, the following features have been reported: bluish-reddish coloration, multicolored "rainbow" pattern (Figure 31.8b), scaly surface, and small brown globules.[30-32] In a study on more than 100 KS lesions from 7 patients, the rainbow pattern was observed in 100% of the cases.[30] It might represent an optic phenomenon due to the interaction of light with the vascular network (diffraction). Some authors suggested that only papular- or nodular-type lesions show the rainbow pattern, which would be completely absent in macular and bullous lesions.[33] However, other authors state that KS lacks any specific feature on dermatoscopy,[34-36] as a similar rainbow phenomenon may also be detected in some non-KS lesions, such as melanoma, stasis dermatitis, lichen planus, hemosiderotic dermatofibroma, and angiosarcoma.[35,37] Although the rainbow pattern may not be specific for KS, dermatoscopic features combined with clinical appearance and patient's history may be helpful in reaching a conclusive diagnosis. Larger studies involving KS and non-KS lesions are required to determine the sensitivity and specificity of the rainbow pattern.

CUTANEOUS MASTOCYTOSIS

Definition

Mastocytosis is a group of disorders characterized by mast cell proliferation and accumulation in one or more organs; the skin is the most commonly involved structure.[38-39]

Epidemiology/Etiopathogenesis

Cutaneous mastocytosis may be present at birth or develop any time thereafter into late adulthood, with no preference for gender or race. The reason for mast cell accumulation in tissues is not yet clear. Specific gene mutations in the proto-oncogene KIT, which encodes a transmembrane tyrosine kinase receptor on mast cells, have been recognized and seem to play a central role in the pathogenesis.

Clinical presentation/Diagnosis

According to World Health Organization (WHO) criteria, the following cutaneous variants were defined: maculopapular cutaneous mastocytosis (urticaria pigmentosa, or UP), diffuse cutaneous mastocytosis, and mastocytoma. There are some less common subtypes, such as nodular, plaque, and telangiectasia type (telangiectasia macularis eruptiva perstans, or TMEP).[39] UP usually begins in childhood but may also affect adults. UP lesions consist of red-brownish maculae, papules, nodules and/or plaques with various sizes; clinical manifestations differ according to the patient's age. In adults the lesions are characterized by red-brownish maculae or slightly elevated papules and vary between 3 and 4 mm in diameter, with symmetrical but random distribution, mainly localized on the trunk and thighs. Involvement in children is usually more extensive, with lesions more hyperpigmented than erythematous and varying between 5 and 15 mm in size (Figure 31.9a). The trunk is the region most commonly affected; the face and scalp are rarely involved. Especially in children, lesions may become erythematous and/or urticated after scratching or rubbing (Darier's sign).[39] Diffuse cutaneous mastocytosis is characterized by mast cell infiltration of the entire skin, which appears yellowish-brown and thickened with a "peau d'orange" aspect.[39] Mastocytoma of skin generally presents before 6 months of age with one or a few (maximum of five) tan-brown nodules mainly located on the distal extremities. TMEP, unlike other forms of cutaneous mastocytosis, affects mainly young adults. The clinical picture is characterized by telangiectasic, brownish-erythematous macules with irregular borders and a diameter between 2 and 6 mm; the chest and limbs are the most frequently involved sites[40] (Figure 31.10a). Darier's sign is absent in most cases.

Dermatoscopy/Videodermatoscopy features

The dermatoscopic pattern of cutaneous mastocytosis varies according to the disease

Miscellaneous Disorders

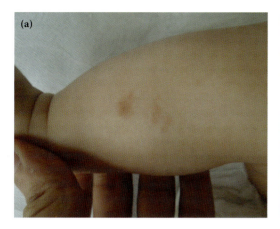
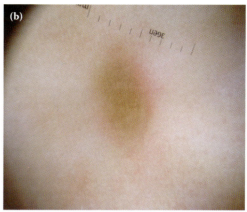

FIGURE 31.9 Mastocytosis. (a) Brownish maculopapules involving the right leg of a child suffering from urticaria pigmentosa. (b) Dermatoscopy of a lesion showing a brownish network; an erythematous halo, due to mechanical stimulation, is also evident (×10).

subtype. One study of 127 patients with cutaneous mastocytosis found that light-brown blot and pigment network (Figure 31.9b) were more prevalent in patients suffering from UP and nodular/plaque subtypes, while reticular vessels (Figure 31.10b) were mostly seen in patients with TMEP and the yellow-orange blot was more prevalent in mastocytoma (and less frequently in nodular mastocytosis).[41] The dermatoscopic patterns observed in different skin lesions in the same patient were similar. Interestingly, the reticular vessels were also seen in UP, and according to the authors, this pattern, together with serum tryptase levels and plaque-type lesions, represented the best combination to predict the need for maintained antimediator therapy.[41] Although the vascular pattern observed in mastocytosis is mainly characterized by thin reticular telangiectasias on a mild erythematous base with sparse vessels dotted throughout,[41] a vascular pattern consisting of thin and tortuous linear vessels associated with fine pigment network and/or homogeneous brownish background may be seen, especially in TMEP.[42] The vessels seen on dermatoscopic examination correspond histologically to dilatation and vascular proliferation associated with the presence of mast cells in the dermis.[41–42] Regarding the pigment network pattern, it is believed that this is due to a

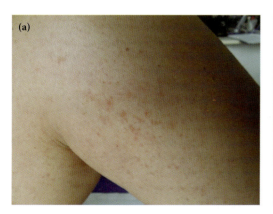
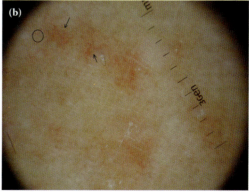

FIGURE 31.10 Mastocytosis. (a) Brownish-erythematous macules involving the left leg of a woman suffering from TMEP. (b) Dermatoscopy showing thin and tortuous linear vessels, some of which intersect to form a network-like structure (arrow), on a brownish background; a few dotted vessels are also evident (circle) (×10).

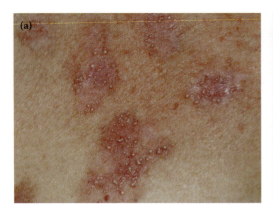 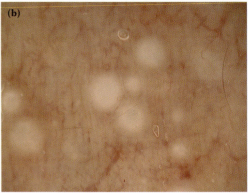

FIGURE 31.11 (a) Secondary milia in a patient affected by bullous pemphigoid. (b) Dermatoscopy showing the presence of roundish structures with a homogeneous yellowish-white coloration (×30).

high concentration of mast cell growth factor that stimulates melanocyte proliferation and melanogenesis, which leads to hyperpigmentation of basal keratinocytes.[41,43]

MILIA

Definition

Milia are benign, asymptomatic, superficial small whitish cysts. They may occur spontaneously (primary milia) or may be secondary to various processes (secondary milia).[44]

Epidemiology/Etiopathogenesis

Milia are very common lesions. Primary milia originate from the lower portion of the infundibulum of vellus hairs and are typically seen in infants, although they may also occur in children and adults. In secondary milia, the lesions generally arise following blistering or trauma due to disruption of the sweat ducts. Secondary milia have been described following different cutaneous disorders, among these bullous pemphigoid (Figure 31.11a), inherited and acquired epidermolysis bullosa, bullous lichen planus, porphyria cutanea tarda, contact dermatitis, and burns.[45–46] They have also been reported following the use of potent topical corticosteroids and from dermabrasion, radiotherapy, and tattoos.[47]

Clinical presentation/Diagnosis

Clinically, milia appear as asymptomatic, superficial, uniform, pearly white to yellowish, dome-shaped papules measuring 1–2 mm in diameter, occurring especially on the face. They may be also found on the mucosa (Epstein pearls) and palate (Bohn nodules). The histological features of milia are identical to those of epidermoid cysts, although the lesions are smaller. They are usually localized in the superficial dermis, and a complete stratified squamous epithelium with keratin is arranged in concentric laminated layers.

Generally, no laboratory or instrumental investigations are needed for milia, as the diagnosis is clinical.

Dermatoscopy/Videodermatoscopy features

In doubtful cases (posttraumatic and/or secondary milia) dermatoscopy may be helpful for the differential diagnosis with clinically similar lesions such as molluscum contagiosum and viral warts. Dermatoscopic examination of milia, both primary and secondary, shows in all cases the same repetitive pattern consisting of the presence of homogeneously yellowish-white coloration over the whole area (Figure 31.11b).

REFERENCES

1. Powell JJ, Wojnarowska F: Lichen sclerosus. *Lancet.* 1999;353:1777–83.
2. Fistarol SK, Itin PH. Diagnosis and treatment of lichen sclerosus: An update. *Am J Clin Dermatol.* 2013;14:27–47.
3. Chan I, Oyama N, Neill SM, et al. Characterization of IgG autoantibodies to extracellular matrix protein 1 in lichen sclerosus. *Clin Exp Dermatol.* 2004;29:499–504.
4. Garrido-Ríos AA, Alvarez-Garrido H, Sanz-Muñoz C, et al. Dermoscopy of extragenital lichen sclerosus. *Arch Dermatol.* 2009;145:1468.
5. Shim WH, Jwa SW, Song M, et al. Diagnostic usefulness of dermatoscopy in differentiating lichen sclerous et atrophicus from morphea. *J Am Acad Dermatol.* 2012;66:690–91.
6. Larre Borges A, Tiodorovic-Zivkovic D, Lallas A, et al. Clinical, dermoscopic and histopathologic features of genital and extragenital lichen sclerosus. *J Eur Acad Dermatol Venereol.* 2013;27:1433–39.
7. Lacarrubba F, Pellacani G, Verzì AE, et al. Extragenital lichen sclerosus: Clinical, dermoscopic, confocal microscopy and histologic correlations. *J Am Acad Dermatol.* 2015;72(1 Suppl):S50–52.
8. Saxton-Daniels S, Jacobe HT. Morphea. In: Goldsmith LA, Katz SI, Gilchrest BA, Paller AS, Leffell DJ, Wolff K, eds. *Fitzpatrick's Dermatology in General Medicine.* 8th ed. New York: McGraw-Hill, 2012:692–701.
9. Campione E, Paternò EJ, Diluvio L, et al. Localized morphea treated with imiquimod 5% and dermoscopic assessment of effectiveness. *J Dermatol Treat.* 2009;20:10–13.
10. Leitenberger JJ, Cayce RL, Haley RW, et al. Distinct autoimmune syndromes in morphea: A review of 245 adult and pediatric cases. *Arch Dermatol.* 2009;145:545–50.
11. Succaria F, Kurban M, Kibbi AG, Abbas O. Clinicopathological study of 81 cases of localized and systemic scleroderma. *J Eur Acad Dermatol Venereol.* 2013;27:e191–96.
12. Daoud MS, Pittelkow MR. Lichen nitidus. In: Goldsmith LA, Katz SI, Gilchrest BA, Paller AS, Leffell DJ, Wolff K, eds. *Fitzpatrick's Dermatology in General Medicine.* 8th ed. New York: McGraw-Hill; 2012:312–16.
13. Leung AK, Ng J. Generalized lichen nitidus in identical twins. *Case Rep Dermatol Med.* 2012;2012:982084.
14. Veasey JV, Framil VM, Nadal SR, et al. Genital warts: Comparing clinical findings to dermatoscopic aspects, in vivo reflectance confocal features and histopathologic exam. *An Bras Dermatol.* 2014;89:137–40.
15. Morales A, Puig S, Zaballos P, Malvehy J. Dermoscopy of molluscum contagiosum. *Arch Dermatol.* 2005;141:1644.
16. Burge S, Hovnanian A. Acantholytic disorders of the skin. In: Goldsmith LA, Katz SI, Gilchrest BA, Paller AS, Leffell DJ, Wolff K, eds. *Fitzpatrick's Dermatology in General Medicine.* 8th ed. New York: McGraw-Hill, 2012:550–57.
17. Vázquez-López F, Lopez-Escobar M, Maldonado-Seral C, et al. The handheld dermoscope improves the recognition of giant pseudocomedones in Darier's disease. *J Am Acad Dermatol.* 2004;50:454–55.
18. Errichetti E, Stinco G, Lacarrubba F, Micali G. Dermoscopy of Darier's disease. *J Eur Acad Dermatol,* in press.
19. Giacomel J, Zalaudek I, Argenziano G. Dermatoscopy of Grover's disease and solitary acantholytic dyskeratoma shows a brown, star-like pattern. *Australas J Dermatol.* 2012;53:315–16.
20. Micali G, Lacarrubba F. Augmented diagnostic capability using videodermatoscopy on selected infectious and non-infectious penile growths. *Int J Dermatol.* 2011;50:1501–5.
21. Ozeki M, Saito R, Tanaka M. Dermoscopic features of pearly penile papules. *Dermatology.* 2008;217:21–22.
22. Diaz Gonzales JM, Martinez Luna E, Pena Romero A, et al. Vestibular papillomatosis as a normal vulvar anatomical condition. *Dermatol Online J.* 2013;19:20032.
23. Wollina U, Verma S. Vulvar vestibular papillomatosis. *Indian J Dermatol Venereol Leprol.* 2010;76:270–72.
24. Kim SH, Seo SH, Ko HC, et al. The use of dermatoscopy to differentiate vestibular papillae, a normal variant of the female external genitalia, from condyloma acuminata. *J Am Acad Dermatol.* 2009;60:353–55.
25. Radu O, Pantanowitz L. Kaposi sarcoma. *Arch Pathol Lab Med.* 2013;137:289–94.
26. Fatahzadeh M. Kaposi sarcoma: Review and medical management update. *Oral Surg Oral Med Oral Pathol Oral Radiol.* 2012;113:2–16.
27. North PE, Kincannon J. Vascular neoplasms and neoplastic-like proliferations. In: Bolognia JL, Jorizo JL, Rapini LP. *Dermatology.* 2nd ed. Mosby Elsevier, 2008:1771–94.

28. Ruocco E, Ruocco V, Tornesello ML, et al. Kaposi's sarcoma: Etiology and pathogenesis, inducing factors, causal associations, and treatments: facts and controversies. *Clin Dermatol.* 2013;31:413–22.
29. Uldrick TS, Whitby D. Update on KSHV epidemiology, Kaposi sarcoma pathogenesis, and treatment of Kaposi sarcoma. *Cancer Lett.* 2011;305:150–62.
30. Cheng S-T, Ke C-LK, Lee C-H, et al. Rainbow pattern in Kaposi's sarcoma under polarized dermoscopy: a dermoscopic pathological study. *Br J Dermatol.* 2009;160:801–9.
31. Hu SC, Ke C-L, Lee C-H, et al. Dermoscopy of Kaposi's sarcoma: Areas exhibiting the multicoloured "rainbow pattern." *J Eur Acad Dermatol Venereol.* 2009;23:1128–32.
32. Grazzini M, Stanganelli I, Rossari S, et al. Dermoscopy, confocal laser microscopy, and hi-tech evaluation of vascular skin lesions: Diagnostic and therapeutic perspectives. *Dermatol Ther.* 2012;25:297–303.
33. Satta R, Fresi L, Cottoni F. Dermoscopic rainbow pattern in Kaposi's sarcoma lesions: Our experience. *Arch Dermatol.* 2012;148:1207–8.
34. Krischer J, Braun RP, Toutous-Trellu L, et al. Kaposi's sarcoma: A new approach of lesional follow-up using epiluminescent light microscopy. *Dermatology.* 1999;198:420–22.
35. Vázquez-López F, García-García B, Rajadhyaksha M, Marghoob AA. Dermoscopic rainbow pattern in non-Kaposi sarcoma lesions. *Br J Dermatol.* 2009;161:474–75.
36. Coates D, Bowling J. Dermoscopy is not always helpful in the diagnosis of vascular lesions. *Australas J Dermatol.* 2010;51:292–94.
37. Oiso N, Matsuda H, Kawada A. Various colour gradations as a dermatoscopic feature of cutaneous angiosarcoma of the scalp. *Australas J Dermatol.* 2013;54:36–38.
38. Valent P. Diagnostic evaluation and classification of mastocytosis. *Immunol Allergy Clin North Am.* 2006;26:515–34.
39. Maluf LC, Barros JA, Machado Filho CD. Mastocytosis. *An Bras Dermatol.* 2009;84:213–25.
40. Costa DL, Moura HH, Rodrigues R, et al. Telangiectasia macularis eruptiva perstans: A rare form of adult mastocytosis. *J Clin Aesthet Dermatol.* 2011;4:52–54.
41. Vano-Galvan S, Alvarez-Twose I, De las Heras E, et al. Dermoscopic features of skin lesions in patients with mastocytosis. *Arch Dermatol.* 2011;147:932–40.
42. Unterstell N, Lavorato FG, Nery NS, et al. Dermatoscopic findings in telangiectasia macularis eruptiva perstans. *An Bras Dermatol.* 2013;88:643–45.
43. Miller MD, Nery NS, Gripp AC, et al. Dermatoscopic findings of urticaria pigmentosa. *An Bras Dermatol.* 2013;88:986–88.
44. Berk DR, Bayliss SJ. Milia: A review and classification. *J Am Acad Dermatol.* 2008;59:1050–63.
45. Hisa T, Goto Y, Taniguchi S, et al. Postbullous milia. *Australas J Dermatol.* 1996;37:153–54.
46. Lucke T, Fallowfield M, Burden D. Lichen planus associated with milia. *Clin Exp Dermatol.* 1999;24:266–69.
47. Cohen BH. Prevention of postdermabrasion milia. *J Dermatol Surg Oncol.* 1988;14:1301.

32 Photodamaged and aged skin

Anne-Sophie Brillouet and Michael D. Southall

DERMATOSCOPY AND SKIN GLYPHICS

Human skin is not a flat, dimensionless surface. It is traversed by a microstructure network of irregularly geometric-shaped patterns called glyphics. In 1926 Harold Cummins coined the name *dermatoglyphics* to describe what had previously been referred to as epidermal ridge configurations, or "skin carvings."[1]

Advances in the field of dermatoscopy have permitted a much more thorough and exhaustive examination of dermatoglyphics than was possible when Harold Cummins conducted his visual assessments of skin. Dermatoscopic studies of dermatoglyphics have shown that glyphic patterns differ based on the region of the body where the skin patterns are located. The glyphic patterns on the palms and soles of feet consist of ridges that form loops, and arches that contribute to the patterns widely recognized in fingerprinting.[2] In contrast, in glabrous skin, the glyphic structures consist of polygonal forms such as trapezoids, triangles, and quadrangles. These polygonal forms manifest as plateaus and furrows across the skin surface, sometimes also referred to as microreliefs (Figure 32.1).

Dermatoscopy can be useful for examining dermatoglyphics in different skin sites across the body to investigate the appearance of glyphics. A dermatoscopic examination of regional skin sites from a single individual clearly shows differences in the appearance of skin glyphics (Figure 32.2). Skin regions that would be considered photoprotected, such as the upper leg (thigh) and abdomen, show distinct glyphic patterns with polygonal forms forming the expected plateaus and furrows across the skin surface. In the same individual, regions of skin that would be expected to be exposed to some sun exposure, such as the upper dorsal arm and dorsal hand, present with less distinct polygonal forms and less defined plateaus and furrows. In contrast, photoexposed regions of skin, such as the cheek and lower outer leg, clearly show a loss of dermatoglyphic patterns of the skin; the primary lines of the polygonal forms appear deeper and wider, and the secondary lines appear flatter and may even disappear from the skin. In regions of the skin that may receive the most sun exposure, such as the cheeks, the glyphics are absent.

Another study quantitated the ridge density in the glyph plateaus and found that abdominal skin had a higher density of ridges compared to the forearm, again suggesting that photoexposure can greatly impact the appearance of skin glyphs.[3] Taken together, the dermatoglyphic patterns suggest that glyphs may be correlated to photoexposure; it is unclear whether the loss of glyphic patterns is a result of intrinsic aging or extrinsic (photodamage/photoaging).

SKIN MICROGLYPHICS AS A FUNCTION OF AGING

Dermal photoaging is manifested primarily as the loss and disorganization of collagen fibrils including loss of fibrillar collagens (I and III in the dermis, and VII anchoring fibrils at the dermo-epidermal junction [DEJ])[4–6] and the accumulation of abundant abnormal amorphous elastin fibers containing material, namely elastosis, at the junction of papillary and reticular dermis.[7] Sun-exposure-increased elastin fibers are abnormally located in the areas previously held by collagen.[8] The oxytalan fibers at the DEJ are markedly reduced, and discrete microfibrillar bundles are rarely observed in photoaged skin.[9] The loss of elastic fiber integrity leads to a progressive reduction of skin elasticity and manifests as skin wrinkles. Photoaged skin has reduced levels of hyaluronic acid and elevated levels of chondroitin sulphate proteoglycans.[10] The decreased hyaluronic acid content in the dermis during photoaging and the subsequent

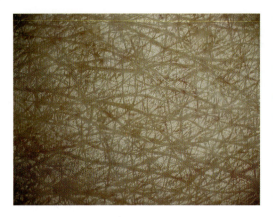

FIGURE 32.1 Dermatoscopy of skin glyphic: the polygonal forms comprise the plateaus and furrows patterns seen across the skin surface (×50, parallel-polarized lens).

reduced water binding capacity skin can also contribute to skin wrinkling and altered elasticity. While the biology of photoaging in the epidermis and dermis has been well documented, few studies have examined the changes in skin glyphics during the aging process.

Dermatoscopy has been used to investigate the differences in skin glyphics between infants (6–24 months old) and adults (25–46 years old). The skin glyphic pattern in infants was more dense and more defined than that in adults, with polygonal forms forming the familiar plateaus and furrows and the "island" regions defined by a glyph more rounded.[11] Interestingly, however, the depth of the skin glyphics was similar in infants and adults, although these results did not determine whether the change in skin glyphics was a result of intrinsic or extrinsic aging. Various quantification methods have been published for images of skin glyphics obtained from dermatoscopy as a way to correlate skin glyphics with skin aging. Zou and co-workers calculated the mean area of skin glyphics formed by the primary and secondary lines and demonstrated a significant correlation between age and skin glyphics,[12] although this was calculated using dermatoscopic images from only two body sites.

A more comprehensive dermatoscopic study of skin glyphics acquired from the same region of skin of different-age patients was conducted to determine whether the change in glyphics was due to intrinsic or extrinsic aging. Photoprotected (abdomen and upper leg) and photoexposed (hand

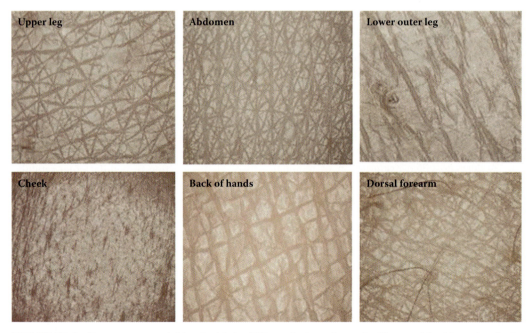

FIGURE 32.2 Dermatoscopy of skin glyphic in different body regions of a 33-year-old subject: the glyphics pattern is very distinct in photoexposed skin sites compared to photoprotected skin sites (×50, parallel-polarized lens).

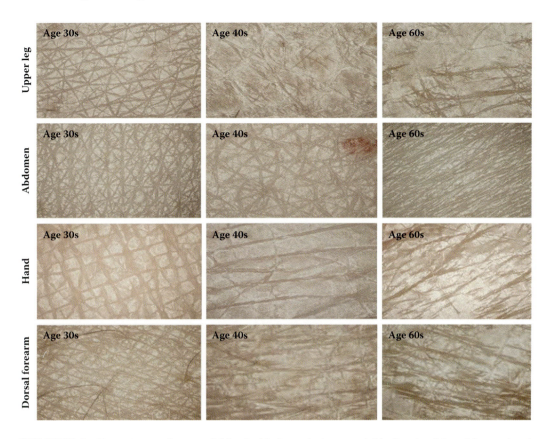

FIGURE 32.3 Dermatoscopy images of skin glyphic from photoexposed skin (hand and dorsal forearm) and photoprotected skin (upper leg and abdomen) from subjects in various age groups: skin glyphic patterns show both the accelerated loss of microstructure in photoexposed skin sites compared to photoprotected skin sites and the loss of microstructure from intrinsic aging (×50, parallel-polarized lens).

and dorsal forearm) sites were acquired from individuals aged 30s, 40s, and 60s. A dermatoscopic examination of regional skin sites from different-aged individuals clearly shows that the appearance of glyphs is affected by both intrinsic and extrinsic aging (Figures 32.2 and 32.3). The glyphic pattern of photoexposed skin (hand and dorsal forearm) sites clearly shows an earlier chronological age loss of glyphics than photoprotected sites. In contrast, photoprotected sites such as the abdomen and upper leg show that a decrease in the appearance of glyphic patterns does occur, but it occurs at a later age than does the loss of glyphic patterns in photoexposed skin. The results of dermatoscopy studies suggest that dermatoglyphics on skin can be affected by both extrinsic and intrinsic aging, and that skin glyphics disappear earlier in aging due to extrinsic aging than due to intrinsic aging. Thus, skin glyphics may be a surrogate marker for premature skin aging.

EVALUATING SKIN GLYPHIC CHANGES WITH EMOLLIENT TREATMENT

In addition to investigating age and skin region changes in dermatoglyphics, dermatoscopy can also be used to evaluate the effects of topical emollient therapy on skin microrelief and skin health.

Skin moisturization is significantly decreased when the skin is damaged, and skin repair can be dependent on retarding the loss of moisture from the skin. The unique structure of the stratum corneum of the skin contributes to its function as a barrier to water loss and the external harsh environment. Injury to this barrier by the environment, UV exposure, common irritants, and age, with the resulting loss of water from the skin, is an important cause of the development of dry skin.

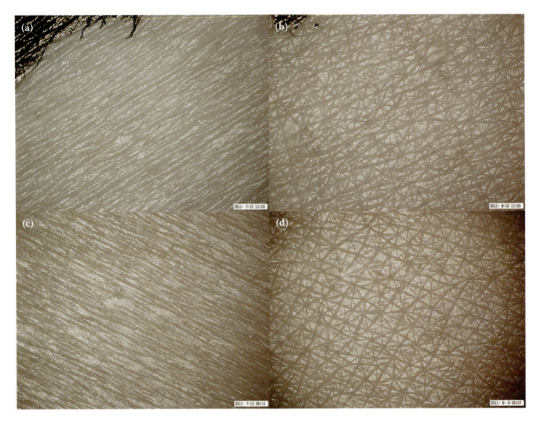

FIGURE 32.4 Dermatoscopy images of skin glyphics from photoexposed skin at baseline (left image, a and c) and after 4 weeks of treatment with an emollient lotion (right image, b and d): restoration of the skin glyphic patterns (×50, parallel-polarized lens).

Emollients or moisturizers help increase the hydration of the skin and may indirectly contribute to the skin barrier repair process. Emollient therapy is widely used in various dermatologic and cosmetic skin treatments to replace natural skin lipids, to cover tiny fissures in the skin barrier, and to provide a soothing, protective skin barrier film.[13] Emollients slow evaporation of the skin's moisture, thereby maintaining hydration and improving the appearance and tactile properties of dry and aging skin. Different classes of emollients or moisturizers are based on their mechanism of action, including humectants and occlusives. Humectants attract and bind water in the stratum corneum from the dermis and can also mimic the role of natural hydrophilic components in the stratum corneum. Humectant molecules include amino acids, lactic acids, alpha hydroxy acids, propylene glycol, glycerin, and urea. Some of these agents are the components of the skin's natural moisturizing factor (NMF), a collection of water-soluble compounds that are only found in the stratum corneum and absorb water from the atmosphere and combine it with their own water content, allowing the outermost layers of the stratum corneum to stay hydrated despite exposure to the elements.[14] Because NMF components are water soluble, they are easily leached from the cells with water contact—which is why repeated contact with water actually makes the skin drier. The lipid layer surrounding the corneocyte helps seal the corneocyte layer to prevent loss of NMF. Occlusive agents increase the skin's moisture content by providing a hydrophobic barrier over the skin. Occlusives, such as petrolatum, form an occlusive film on the skin that reduces the transepidermal water lost (TEWL) by preventing evaporation of water from the stratum corneum.[15] These agents can diffuse into the intracellular lipid domains and may also help to restore the lipid barrier of the skin.

A dermatoscopic examination of regional skin sites from subjects using a topical emollient lotion clearly shows differences in the appearance of skin glyphics (Figure 32.4). Images of skin glyphics obtained prior to emollient therapy clearly show a loss of dermatoglyphic pattern of the skin; the primary lines appear deep and wide and the secondary lines appear flatter or are absent. Subjects used a topical emollient lotion for 4 weeks, and the same site was again imaged using dermatoscopy. Treatment with an emollient lotion restored the appearance of the skin glyphics with the primary lines of the polygonal forms forming the familiar plateaus and furrows, and in several subjects the secondary lines reappeared after being absent in the baseline images.

ROLE OF SKIN GLYPHICS AS A RESERVOIR FOR EMOLLIENTS AND OTHER TOPICAL AGENTS

While it is unclear whether there is a physiological purpose for skin glyphics, several theories have been proposed. First, skin glyphics may increase the surface area of skin, thereby providing more interface for thermoregulation.[2] Other theories suggest that skin glyphics may act as a conduit on the skin surface. Zhang and colleagues investigated the distribution of oleic acid on the skin using infrared microscopy. After topical administration on the skin, oleic acid was found to spread laterally across the skin, and the pattern of the distribution was correlated with glyphics regions on skin.[16] The skin glyphics were proposed to act as skin channels for lateral diffusion across the skin surface. In addition, it was proposed that skin glyphics themselves might act as reservoirs for emollients and other topical agents applied to the skin. Thus in photoexposed or aged skin, where the skin glyphics are absent, the lack of skin glyphics may impair skin transport and skin reservoir effect and thereby contribute to age-dependent skin dryness.

CONCLUSION

Dermatoscopy has been shown to be a useful resource for researchers investigating clinical and cosmetic applications in skin care.[17] Additional applications of dermatoscopy show it to be an extremely valuable tool for examining skin expression of dermatoglyphics as a function of age and photoexposure. The ability to acquire high-resolution images of the skin surface has enabled researchers to investigate and follow changes in the appearance of dermatoglyphics during topical treatments.

REFERENCES

1. Cummins H. Dermatoglyphics: Significant patternings of the body surface. *Yale J Biol Med*. 1946;18:551–65.
2. El Gammal C, Kligman AM, El Gammal S. Anatomy of the skin surface. In: Wilhelm KP, Elsner P, Berardesca E, Maibach H, eds. *Bioengineering of the Skin: Skin surface Imaging and Analysis*. New York: CRC Press, 2007: 3–16.
3. Oh GN, Yoon JH, Kye HS, et al. 3D reconstruction of skin pathological tissue: The understanding of microrelief pattern and dermal ridge. *Skin Res Technol*. 2014;20:213–17.
4. El-Domyati M, Attia S, Saleh F, et al. Intrinsic aging vs. photoaging: A comparative histopathological, immunohistochemical, and ultrastructural study of skin. *Exp Dermatol*. 2002;11:398–405.
5. Craven NM, Watson RE, Jones CJ, et al. Clinical features of photodamaged human skin are associated with a reduction in collagen VII. *Br J Dermatol*. 1997;137:344–50.
6. Talwar HS, Griffiths CE, Fisher GJ, et al. Reduced type I and type III procollagens in photodamaged adult human skin. *J Invest Dermatol*. 1995;105:285–90.
7. Gilchrest BA, Rogers G. Photoaging. In: Lim H, Soter N, eds. *Clinical Photomedicine*. New York: Marcel Dekker, 1993:95–111.
8. Lewis KG, Bercovitch L, Dill SW, Robinson-Bostom L. Acquired disorders of elastic tissue: Part I. Increased elastic tissue and solar elastotic syndromes. *J Am Acad Dermatol*. 2004;51:1–21.
9. Watson RE, Griffiths CE, Craven NM, et al. Fibrillin-rich microfibrils are reduced in photoaged skin. Distribution at the dermal-epidermal junction. *J Invest Dermatol*. 1999;112:782–87.
10. Bernstein EF, Underhill CB, Hahn PJ, et al. Chronic sun exposure alters both the content and distribution of dermal glycosaminoglycans. *Br J Dermatol*. 1996;135:255–62.
11. Stamatas GN, Nikolovski J, Luedtke MA, et al. Infant skin microstructure assessed in vivo differs from adult skin in organization and at the cellular level. *Pediatr Dermatol*. 2010;27:125–31.

12. Zou Y, Song E, Jin R. Age-dependent changes in skin surface assessed by a novel two-dimensional image analysis. *Skin Res Technol.* 2009;15:399–406.
13. Lodén M, Maibach HI, eds. *Dry Skin and Moisturizers: Chemistry and Function.* New York: CRC Press, 2000.
14. Harding C, Bartolone J, Rawlings, A. Effects of natural moisturizing factor and lactic acid isomers on skin function. In: Loden M, Maibach H, eds. *Dry Skin and Moisturizers; Chemistry and Function.* New York: CRC Press, 2000;229–41.
15. Ghadially R, Halkier-Sorenson L, Elias P. Effects of peterolatum on stratum corneum structure and function. *J Am Acad Dermatol.* 1992;26:387–96.
16. Zhang Q, Saad P, Mao G, et al. Infrared spectroscopic imaging tracks lateral distribution in human stratum corneum. *Pharm Res.* 2014;10:2762–73.
17. Wallo, W. Dermatoscopy in cosmetic applications. In: Micali G, Lacarrubba F, eds. *Dermatoscopy in Clinical Practice: Beyond Pigmented Lesions.* London: Informa Healthcare, 2010;121–26.

Index

A

Actinic keratosis (AK), 151–153
    clinical discrimination, 153
    clinical presentation/diagnosis, 152
    definition, 151
    dermatoscopy/videodermatoscopy features, 152–153
    epidemiology/etiopathogenesis, 151–152
    histopathology, 152
Aged skin, *see* Photodamaged and aged skin
AH, *see* Apocrine hidrocystoma
Alopecia areata, 55–57
Alopecia areata incognita, 57–58
Amelanotic melanomas, 122
Analog videodermatoscopy, 1
Androgenetic alopecia (AGA), 55, 56
Angiokeratoma, 125–126
    clinical presentation/diagnosis, 125
    clinical variants, 125
    definition, 125
    dermatoscopy/videodermatoscopy features, 125–126
    epidemiology/etiopathogenesis, 125
Apocrine hidrocystoma (AH), 141–143
    clinical presentation/diagnosis, 141
    definition, 141
    dermatoscopy/videodermatoscopy features, 141–143
        chrysalis, 142
        "hidrocystoma noir," 143
        pigmentation, 141
        Tyndall phenomenon, 141
    epidemiology/etiopathogenesis, 141
    Schöpf-Schulz-Passarge syndrome, 141
Arboriform vessels, 90, 162

B

Basal cell carcinoma, 33, 71, 134
Black dots, 28, 39, 47, 52, 56–58, 61, 62, 89
Bohn nodules, 176
Bowen's disease (BD), 145–149, 151
    clinical presentation/diagnosis, 145
    definition, 145
    dermatoscopy/videodermatoscopy features, 145–147
        dotted vessels, 147
        "glomerular vessels," 146
        pigmentation, 148
        vascular structures, 146
    epidemiology/etiopathogenesis, 145
    unusual variants, 145
Burrow, 9-13, 23, 31
Bushy capillaries, 70–74, 81, 93, 95

C

Cadaverized hairs, 57–58
Candidiasis, 74
Capillary malformations (CMs), 159–165
    clinical presentation/diagnosis, 159
    definition, 159
    dermatoscopy/videodermatoscopy features, 160–164
        depth-measuring videomicroscope, 163
        dermatoscopic patterns, 160
        hemangiomas, 161, 164
        laser treatment, 161–162, 163
        structures, 160
        vessel types, 160–161
    epidemiology/etiopathogenesis, 159
    gene mutation, 159
    Klippel-Trenaunay syndrome, 159
    Parkes Weber syndrome, 159
    Sturge-Weber syndrome, 159
    vascular malformations, 159
Central centrifugal cicatricial alopecia (CCCA), 61–62
"Chiggers," *see* Trombiculiasis
Chondroitin sulphate proteoglycans, 179
CL, *see* Cutaneous leishmaniasis
Clear cell acanthoma (CCA), 117–120, 122
    clinical presentation/diagnosis, 117
    definition, 117
    dermatoscopy/videodermatoscopy features, 117–119
        characterization, 117
        dermatoscopic pattern, 118
        differential diagnosis, 119
    epidemiology/etiopathogenesis, 117
    ichthyosis, 117
    varicose veins, 117
CLM, *see* Cutaneous larva migrans
CMs, *see* Capillary malformations
Comma hairs, 47, 51
Common urticaria (CU), 87–91
    clinical presentation/diagnosis, 87
    definition, 87
    dermatoscopy/videodermatoscopy features, 88–91
        dermatoscopic semiology, 90
        discrimination between CU and UV, 91
        transient wheals, 89
        vascular structures, 88
    epidemiology/etiopathogenesis, 87
Congenital triangular alopecia, 58
Connective tissue diseases, 93–96
    clinical presentation/diagnosis, 93
    definition, 93
    dermatomyositis, 93
    dermatoscopy/videodermatoscopy features, 93–96
        capillaroscopy, 93
        cutaneous discoid lupus erythematosus, 95
        nailfold capillary microscopy, 93, 94
        Raynaud's phenomenon, 93
        scleroderma pattern, 94
    epidemiology/etiopathogenesis, 93
    lupus erythematosus, 93
    systemic sclerosis, 93
Contact dermatoscopy, 3
Crab lice, 17–19

clinical presentation/diagnosis, 17–18
contamination, 17
definition, 17
dermatoscopy/videodermatoscopy features, 18–19
epidemiology/etiopathogenesis, 17
CS, *see* Cutaneous sarcoidosis
CU, *see* Common urticaria
Cutaneous discoid lupus erythematosus, 95
Cutaneous and genital warts, 39–42
    cutaneous warts, 39–40
        clinical presentation/diagnosis, 39
        common warts, 39, 40
        definition, 39
        dermatoscopy/videodermatoscopy features, 39
        epidemiology/etiopathogenesis, 39
        flat warts, 39, 40
        palmo-plantar warts, 39
        plantar warts, 40
    genital warts, 41–42
        cauliflower-like genital wart, 41
        clinical presentation/diagnosis, 41
        definition, 41
        dermatoscopy/videodermatoscopy features, 42
        differentiation from other genital growths, 42
        epidemiology/etiopathogenesis, 41
        papular genital warts, 41
    human papillomaviruses, 39
    morphological variants, 39
Cutaneous larva migrans (CLM), 31–32
    cases, 32
    cause, 31
    clinical presentation/diagnosis, 31
    definition, 31
    dermatoscopy/videodermatoscopy features, 31–32
    epidemiology/etiopathogenesis, 31
    most common parasite implicated, 31
    pruritus, 31
Cutaneous leishmaniasis (CL), 33–35, 11
    advanced phase, 34
    clinical presentation/diagnosis, 33
    common findings, 33
    definition, 33
    dermatoscopic patterns, 35
    dermatoscopy/videodermatoscopy features, 33–35
    differential diagnosis, 33
    epidemiology/etiopathogenesis, 33
    initial phase, 34
    intracellular protozoa, 33
Cutaneous mastocytosis, 174–176
Cutaneous sarcoidosis (CS), 111

D

Darier's disease (DD), 170–171
Demodex mites, 97
Depth-measuring videomicroscope (DMV), 163
Dermatomyositis, 93
Dermo-epidermal junction (DEJ), 179
Dermo-Image, 3, 4
Digital videodermatoscopy, 1–3
Discoid lupus erythematosus (DLE), 59–60
Dissecting cellulitis of the scalp, 61

Disseminated superficial actinic porokeratosis (DSAP), 137
Doppler ultrasound, 159

E

Eggs, 9–11, 15, 21, 25, 27–29
Epiluminescence light microscopy (ELM), 21
Epstein pearls, 176
Epulis gravidarum, 121
Equipment, 1–7
    analog videodermatoscopy, 1
    classifier, building of, 5
    contact, noncontact, and polarized dermatoscopy, 3
    data storage, 3
    digital videodermatoscopy, 1–3
    follow-up, 3
    instruments for digital dermatoscopy analysis, 6
    resolution, 2
    software, 3–5
Exclamation mark hairs, 57–58

F

Febrile ulceronecrotic Mucha-Habermann disease, 105
Flat warts, 39, 40
Foam cells, 131
Folliculitis decalvans (FD), 60, 61
Fordyce's spots of the penile shaft, 171

G

Genital warts, 41–42
    cauliflower-like genital wart, 41
    clinical presentation/diagnosis, 41
    definition, 41
    dermatoscopy/videodermatoscopy features, 42
    differentiation from other genital growths, 42
    epidemiology/etiopathogenesis, 41
    papular genital warts, 41
Glomerular vessels, 41, 42, 103, 123, 146, 147, 155
Granuloma annulare (GA), 111
Granulomatous rosacea (GR), 111
Granulomatous skin disorders (GSDs), 111–114
    clinical presentation/diagnosis, 111
    cutaneous leishmaniasis, 111
    cutaneous sarcoidosis, 111
    definition, 111
    dermatoscopy/videodermatoscopy features, 111–114
    epidemiology/etiopathogenesis, 111
    granuloma annulare, 111
    granulomatous rosacea, 111
    lupus vulgaris, 111
    necrobiosis lipoidica, 111
    yellow patches, 111

H

Hair diameter diversity, 55, 66
Hair loss and hair shaft disorders, 55–66
    alopecia areata, 55–57
        black dots, 57
        clinical presentations, 55
        dystrophic hairs, 56–57
        features, 57
        yellow dots, 56

alopecia areata incognita, 57–58
androgenetic alopecia, 55, 56
congenital triangular alopecia, 58
dermoscopic patterns in normal and pathological scalp, 56
hair diameter diversity, 55
hair shaft disorders, 62–66
    hair shaft disorders associated with increased fragility, 63
    monilethrix, 63
    pili annulati, 65
    pili torti, 64, 65
    pili trianguli and canaliculi, 65, 66
    trichorrhexis invaginata, 63–64
    trichorrhexis nodosa, 64
normal scalp, 55, 56
scalp examination, 55
scarring alopecia, 58–62
    central centrifugal cicatricial alopecia, 61–62
    dermoscopic features, 58, 59
    discoid lupus erythematosus, 59–60
    dissecting cellulitis of the scalp, 61
    folliculitis decalvans, 60, 61
    lichen planopilaris, 58–59
    traction alopecia, 62
trichotillomania, 58
Head lice, 15–17
    clinical presentation/diagnosis, 15
    definition, 15
    dermatoscopy/videodermatoscopy features, 16–17
    epidemiology/etiopathogenesis, 15
    louse combs, 15
    nits, 15, 16
    pseudo-nit, 16
HIV, 173
Human herpes virus-8 (HHV-8), 173
Human papillomaviruses (HPVs), 39

I

Ichthyosis, 117
IL-1, *see* Interleukin-1
Imagestore for Healthcare, 3, 4
Infectious diseases
    cutaneous and genital warts, 39–42
    molluscum contagiosum, 43–45
    tinea capitis, 47–54
Inflammatory diseases
    common urticaria and urticarial vasculitis, 87–91
    connective tissue diseases, 93–96
    granulomatous skin disorders, 111–114
    lichen planus, 79–85
    pigmented purpuric dermatoses, 101–103
    pityriasis lichenoides, 105–109
    psoriasis, 67–78
    rosacea, 97–99
    Wolf's isotopic response lesions, 114–116
Interleukin-1 (IL-1), 69

J

Juvenile xanthogranuloma, 132

K

Kaposi's sarcoma (KS), 122, 173–174
Keratoacanthoma, 154
Keratosis follicularis, 170
Kerion, 50, 52
KIT (proto-oncogene), 174
Klippel-Trenaunay syndrome, 159

L

Leishmaniasis, *see* Cutaneous leishmaniasis
Lice, 15–19, 24–26
Lichen nitidus (LN), 169–170
Lichen planopilaris (LPP), 58–59
Lichen planus (LP), 79–85
    clinical presentation/diagnosis, 79
    definition, 79
    dermatoscopy/videodermatoscopy features, 80–84
        ashy dermatosis, 84
        clinical value of dermatoscopy, 80
        granular pigment, 80–81, 83
        plaque-psoriasis, 81
    epidemiology/etiopathogenesis, 79
    histopathological picture, 79
    pigmentation, 79
    Wickham striae, 79, 80
Lichen sclerosus (LS), 74, 167–168
LN, *see* Lichen nitidus
Localized scleroderma, 168
Louse combs, 15
LP, *see* Lichen planus
LPP, *see* Lichen planopilaris
Lupus erythematosus, 93
Lupus vulgaris (LV), 111

M

Majocchi's disease, 103
MC, *see* Molluscum contagiosum
Menkes syndrome, 64
Microreliefs, 179
Milia, 176
Mirror software, 3, 4
Miscellaneous disorders, 167–176
    cutaneous mastocytosis, 174–176
        clinical presentation/diagnosis, 174
        definition, 174
        dermatoscopy/videodermatoscopy features, 174–176
        epidemiology/etiopathogenesis, 174
        telangiectasia macularis eruptiva perstans, 174
    Darier's disease, 170–171
        clinical presentation/diagnosis, 170–171
        definition, 170
        dermatoscopy/videodermatoscopy, 171
        epidemiology/etiopathogenesis, 170
        forms, 170
    Fordyce's spots of the penile shaft, 171
        clinical presentation/diagnosis, 171
        definition, 171
        dermatoscopy/videodermatoscopy features, 171
        epidemiology/etiopathogenesis, 171

Kaposi's sarcoma, 173–174
    clinical presentation/diagnosis, 173–174
    clinical variants, 173
    definition, 173
    dermatoscopy/videodermatoscopy features, 174
    epidemiology/etiopathogenesis, 173
    HIV, 173
    human herpes virus-8, 173
lichen nitidus, 169–170
    clinical presentation/diagnosis, 169–170
    definition, 169
    dermatoscopy/videodermatoscopy features, 170
    epidemiology/etiopathogenesis, 169
lichen sclerosus, 167–168
    clinical presentation/diagnosis, 167
    definition, 167
    dermatoscopy/videodermatoscopy features, 167, 168
    epidemiology/etiopathogenesis, 167
milia, 176
    Bohn nodules, 176
    clinical presentation/diagnosis, 176
    definition, 176
    dermatoscopy/videodermatoscopy features, 176
    epidemiology/etiopathogenesis, 176
    Epstein pearls, 176
morphea, 168–169
    clinical presentation/diagnosis, 168–169
    definition, 168
    dermatoscopy/videodermatoscopy features, 169
    epidemiology/etiopathogenesis, 168
pearly penile papules and vestibular papillae, 172–173
    clinical presentation/diagnosis, 172–173
    definition, 172
    dermatoscopy/videodermatoscopy features, 173
    epidemiology/etiopathogenesis, 172
Molluscum contagiosum (MC), 43–45
    clinical presentation/diagnosis, 43
    definition, 43
    dermatoscopy/videodermatoscopy features, 43–45
    epidemiology/etiopathogenesis, 43
    lesions, 43, 44
    papules, 45
    pattern, 43
    vascular structure, 44
    virus subtypes, 43
Monilethrix, 63
Morphea, 168–169
Morse-code hairs, 53
Muir-Torre syndrome, 127, 134
Munro microabscesses, 67

N

Nailfold capillary microscopy, 93, 94
National Rosacea Society Expert Committee (USA), 97
National Television Systems Committee (NTSC), 1
Natural moisturizing factor (NMF), 182
Necrobiosis lipoidica (NL), 111
Netherton disease, 63
Nits, 15–18
Noncontact dermatoscopy, 3

Nonpigmented skin lesions
    actinic keratosis, 151–153
    angiokeratoma, 125–126
    apocrine hidrocystoma, 141–143
    Bowen's disease, 145–149
    clear cell acanthoma, 117–120
    porokeratosis, 137–139
    pyogenic granuloma, 121–124
    sebaceous hyperplasia, 127–129
    squamous cell carcinoma, 151, 154–156
    xanthomatous lesions, 131–135
NTSC, *see* National Television Systems Committee

P

Palmo-plantar psoriasis, 72
Palmo-plantar warts, 39
Parasitoses
    cutaneous larva migrans, 31–32
    cutaneous leishmaniasis, 33–35
    pediculosis, 15–19, 24–26
    scabies, 9–14
    therapeutic monitoring of, 21–26
    trombiculiasis, 37–38
    tungiasis, 27–30
Parkes Weber syndrome, 159
PCR, *see* Polymerase chain reaction
Pearly penile papules (PPP), 172–173
Pediculosis, 15–19
    crab lice, 17–19
        clinical presentation/diagnosis, 17–18
        contamination, 17
        definition, 17
        dermatoscopy/videodermatoscopy features, 18–19
        epidemiology/etiopathogenesis, 17
    head lice, 15–17
        clinical presentation/diagnosis, 15
        definition, 15
        dermatoscopy/videodermatoscopy features, 16–17
        epidemiology/etiopathogenesis, 15
        louse combs, 15
        nits, 15, 16
        pseudo-nit, 16
    therapeutic monitoring of, 24–26
        "choking" the mite, 26
        isolation of adult parasite, 25
        noncontact handheld dermatoscope, 25
        overuse of products, 24
        topical compounds, 24
Perifollicular casts, 52, 55, 59
PG, *see* Pyogenic granuloma
Photodamaged and aged skin, 179–183
    chondroitin sulphate proteoglycans, 179
    dermatoscopy and skin glyphics, 179
    dermo-epidermal junction, 179
    emollients and other topical agents, role of skin glyphics as reservoir for, 183
    epidermal ridge configurations, 179
    evaluating skin glyphic changes with emollient treatment, 181–183
    microreliefs, 179
    natural moisturizing factor, 182
    occlusive agents, 182
    oxytalan fibers, 179

Index

photoprotected sites, 181
quantification methods, 180
"skin carvings," 179
skin elasticity, reduction of, 179
skin microglyphics as function of aging, 179–181
transepidermal water lost, 182
Pigmented purpuric dermatoses (PPDs), 101–103
  clinical presentation/diagnosis, 101
  definition, 101
  dermatoscopy/videodermatoscopy features, 101–103
  epidemiology/etiopathogenesis, 101
  Majocchi's disease, 103
  purpura of Doucas and Kapetanakis, 101, 102
  purpura of Gougerot and Blum, 102
  Schamberg's disease, 101, 102
  triggering factors, 101
Pili annulati, 65
Pili torti, 64, 65
Pili trianguli and canaliculi, 65, 66
Pityriasis lichenoides (PL), 105–109
  clinical presentation/diagnosis, 105–106
  definition, 105
  dermatoscopy/videodermatoscopy features, 106–108
  epidemiology/etiopathogenesis, 105
  histopathology, 106
  lesions, 105
  pityriasis lichenoides chronica, 105
  pityriasis lichenoides et varioliformis acuta, 105, 106
Pityriasis lichenoides chronica (PLC), 105
Pityriasis lichenoides et varioliformis acuta (PLEVA), 105, 106
Plantar warts, 40
Plaque psoriasis, 68, 69, 81
Polarized dermatoscopy, 3
Polymerase chain reaction (PCR), 41
Porokeratosis, 137–139
  clinical presentation/diagnosis, 137
  clinical variants, 137
  definition, 137
  dermatoscopy/videodermatoscopy features, 137–139
    "pseudo network," 138
    uncommon structures, 138
    white track, 137
  disseminated superficial actinic porokeratosis, 137
  epidemiology/etiopathogenesis, 137
  superficial, 137
PPDs, see Pigmented purpuric dermatoses
PPP, see Pearly penile papules
Psoriasis, 67–78
  clinical presentation/diagnosis, 67–69
    interleukin-1, 69
    lesions, 67
    microvasculature, 69
    Munro microabscesses, 67
    phases, 67
    plaque psoriasis, 68, 69
    tumor necrosis factor-alpha, 69
    vascular endothelial growth factor, 69
  definition, 67
  dermatoscopy/videodermatoscopy features, 69–76
    active lichen planus lesions, 82
    bushy capillaries, 70
    candidiasis, 74
    dermatoscopic semiology, 81
    genital psoriasis, 73
    lichen sclerosus, 74
    nonpsoriatic balanitis, 74
    palmo-plantar psoriasis, 72
    psoriatic balanitis, 73, 75
    scalp psoriasis, 74, 76
    seborrheic dermatitis, 74
    study, 71
    videocapillaroscopy, 69
    Zoon balanitis, 74, 75
  epidemiology/etiopathogenesis, 67
  therapeutic monitoring of, 76–77
Pubic lice infestation, 17
Pyogenic granuloma (PG), 121–124
  clinical presentation/diagnosis, 121
  definition, 121
  dermatoscopy/videodermatoscopy features, 121–124
    amelanotic melanomas, 122
    basal cell carcinomas, 122
    clear cell acanthomas, 122
    Kaposi's sarcomas, 122
    solitary angiokeratomas, 122
    structures associated with lesion, 121
    ulceration, 123
  differentiation, 121
  epidemiology/etiopathogenesis, 121
  epulis gravidorum, 121
  gingival lesion, 121

R

Raynaud's phenomenon (RP), 93
Reticulohistiocytoma, 133
Rosacea, 97–99
  activation of innate immunity, 97
  clinical presentation/diagnosis, 97
  definition, 97
  dermatoscopy/videodermatoscopy features, 97–99
    facial rosacea, 98
    handheld dermatoscopy, 98, 99
    polygonal net, 97
    videocapillaroscopy, 98, 99
  epidemiology/etiopathogenesis, 97

S

Scabies, 9–14
  clinical presentation/diagnosis, 9–10
  definition, 9
  dermatoscopy/videodermatoscopy features, 10–13
    advantages of dermatoscopy, 11
    comparative study, 10
    cost of devices, 12
    epiluminescence microscopy, 10
    indirect contamination, 13
    magnification, 11
    mite viability, 12
  differential diagnosis, 9
  epidemiology/etiopathogenesis, 9
  standard technique for diagnosis, 9

therapeutic monitoring of, 21–23
    epiluminescence light microscopy, 21
    permethrin cream formulation, 23
    pruritus, 21
    stereo epiluminescence microscope, 23
    topical treatment, 23
Scalp psoriasis, 74, 76
Scalp ringworm, *see* Tinea capitis
Scarring alopecia, 58–62
SCC, *see* Squamous cell carcinoma
Schamberg's disease, 101, 102
Schöpf-Schulz-Passarge syndrome, 141
Sebaceous hyperplasia (SH), 127–129
  clinical presentation/diagnosis, 127
  definition, 127
  dermatoscopy/videodermatoscopy features, 127–129
    "bonbon toffee sign," 127, 128
    "cumulus sign," 127
    vascular structures, 129
  epidemiology/etiopathogenesis, 127
  Muir-Torre syndrome, 127
Seborrheic dermatitis, 74
Sign of the setting sun, 133
Solitary angiokeratomas, 122
Solitary epithelioid histiocytoma, 133
Spitz nevus, 134
Squamous cell carcinoma (SCC), 151, 154–156
  clinical presentation/diagnosis, 154
  dermatoscopy/videodermatoscopy features, 154–156
    keratin masses, 155
    poorly differentiated, 155
    vascular structures, 155
  epidemiology/etiopathogenesis, 154
  keratoacanthoma, 154
  recurrence rate of, 154
  subtypes, 154
Sturge-Weber syndrome (SWS), 159
Systemic sclerosis (SSc), 93

T

Telangiectasia, 33, 34, 59, 97, 98, 101, 123, 129, 138, 141, 142, 159, 167, 168, 174, 175
Telangiectasia macularis eruptiva perstans (TMEP), 174
TEWL, *see* Transepidermal water lost
Tinea capitis (TC), 47–54
  black dot type, 50
  clinical presentation/diagnosis, 47
  comma hairs, 47, 51
  definition, 47
  dermatoscopic features, 48
  dermatoscopy/videodermatoscopy features, 47–53
  epidemiology/etiopathogenesis, 47
  hair invasion types, 47
  high magnification videodermatoscopy, 52
  kerion, 50, 52
  Morse-code hairs, 53
  scaly type, 48, 49
  UV-enhanced trichoscopy, 52
  zigzag hairs, 51, 53
TNF-α, *see* Tumor necrosis factor-alpha

Traction alopecia, 62
Transepidermal water lost (TEWL), 182
Trichorrhexis invaginata, 63–64
Trichorrhexis nodosa, 64
Trichoscan, 5
Trichoscopy, UV-enhanced, 52
Trichotillomania, 58
Trombiculiasis, 37–38
  clinical presentation/diagnosis, 37
  definition, 37
  dermatoscopy/videodermatoscopy features, 37–38
  epidemiology/etiopathogenesis, 37
  immune inflammatory response, 37
  larval stage of mite, 38
  management, 38
  misdiagnosis of, 37
  subjects at risk, 37
  wheals and papules, 38
Tumor necrosis factor-alpha (TNF-α), 69
Tungiasis, 27–30
  clinical presentation/diagnosis, 27–28
  definition, 27
  dermatoscopy/videodermatoscopy features, 28–29
  differential diagnosis, 28
  epidemiology/etiopathogenesis, 27
  histopathic examination, 28
  penetration of the skin, 27
  procedure to remove flea, 29
Tyndall phenomenon, 141

U

Ultraviolet-enhanced trichoscopy, 52
Urticarial vasculitis (UV), 87–91
  clinical presentation/diagnosis, 87
  definition, 87
  dermatoscopy/videodermatoscopy features, 88–91
    dermatoscopic semiology, 90
    discrimination between CU and UV, 91
    lesions, 91
    purpuric structures, 89
    vascular structures, 88
  epidemiology/etiopathogenesis, 87

V

Varicella-zoster virus infection, 114
Varicose veins, 117
Vascular endothelial growth factor (VEGF), 69
Vascular malformations (VMs), 159
Vellus hairs, 52, 55–60, 62, 66, 176
Vestibular papillae (VP), 172–173
Videocapillaroscopy (VCP), 69
Videodermatoscopy, equipment for, 1–7
  analog videodermatoscopy, 1
  classifier, building of, 5
  contact, noncontact, and polarized dermatoscopy, 3
  data storage, 3
  digital videodermatoscopy, 1–3

Index

follow-up, 3
instruments for digital dermatoscopy analysis, 6
resolution, 2
software, 3–5

W

Warts, *see* Cutaneous and genital warts
White collarette, 121-123
White dots, 55–57, 60, 62
Wickham striae (WS), 79, 80, 114
Wolf's isotopic response (WIR) lesions, 114–116
    clinical presentation/diagnosis, 114
    definition, 114
    dermatoscopy/videodermatoscopy features, 114–115
    differential dermatoscopic patterns in post-herpetic WIR lesions, 114
    epidemiology/etiopathogenesis, 114
    pathological mechanisms, 114
    varicella-zoster virus infection, 114

X

Xanthomatous lesions, 131–135
    clinical presentation/diagnosis, 131–133
        diffuse flat normolipidemic xanthomas, 131
        eruptive papular xanthomas, 131
        juvenile xanthogranuloma, 132
        reticulohistiocytoma, 133
        solitary epithelioid histiocytoma, 133
        syndromes associated with skin xanthomas, 132
        tuberous xanthomas, 131
        xanthelasms, 131
        xanthomization, 133
    definition, 131
    dermatoscopy/videodermatoscopy features, 133–135
        basal cell carcinomas, 134
        Bowen's disease, 134
        juvenile xanthogranuloma, 133
        Muir-Torre syndrome, 134
        reticulohistiocytoma, 133
        sign of the setting sun, 133
        Spitz nevus, 134
        xanthomized dermatofibroma, 134
    epidemiology/etiopathogenesis, 131
    foam cells, 131

Y

Yellow dots, 52, 55–58, 61

Z

Zigzag hairs, 51, 53
Zoon balanitis, 74, 75